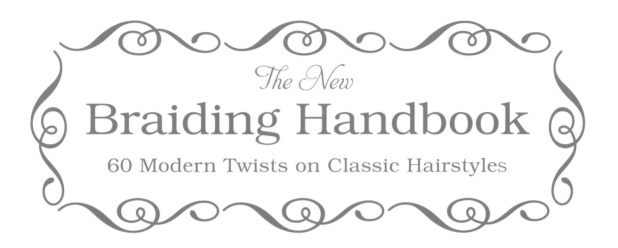

The New
Braiding Handbook
60 Modern Twists on Classic Hairstyles

-Abby Smith-

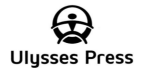

Ulysses Press

Published in the U.S. by
Ulysses Press
P.O. Box 3440
Berkeley, CA 94703
www.ulyssespress.com

ISBN: 978-1-61243-296-0
Library of Congress Control Number 2013957407

Printed in the United States by Bang Printing

10 9 8 7 6 5

Acquisitions Editor: Katherine Furman
Editor: Melanie Gold
Proofreader: Mary Hern
Design and layout: Ashley Prine
Indexer: Jay Kreider, J S Editorial
Cover photograph: Abby Smith

Distributed by Publishers Group West

Contents

Contents

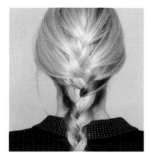

*Basic French
Braid, page 28*

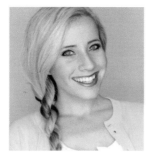

Rope Braid, page 30

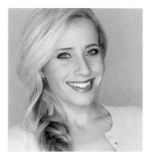

*Alternative Braid,
page 31*

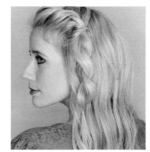

*Falling Bohemian
Twist, page 32*

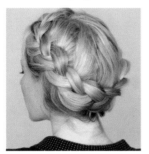

*Bohemian Crown,
page 34*

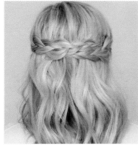

*Braided Crown,
page 36*

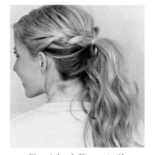

*Braided Ponytail,
page 37*

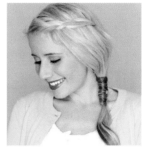

*Chinese Staircase
Stitch, page 38*

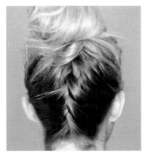

*French Braided
Topknot, page 40*

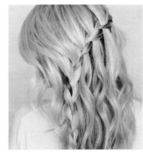

*Waterfall Braid,
page 42*

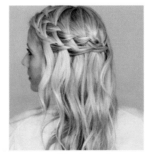

*Double Braids,
page 44*

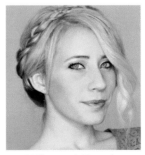

*Milkmaid Braids,
page 46*

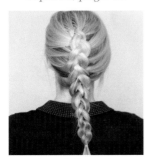

*Dutch French
Braid, page 48*

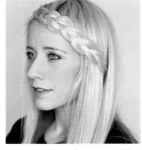

Lace Braid, page 50

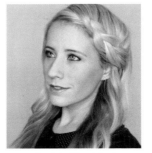

*Dutch Braided
Headband, page 52*

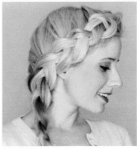

*Side Dutch Braid,
page 53*

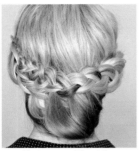

Princess Braids,
page 54

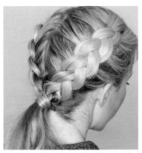

Double-Dutch Pigtail
Braids, page 56

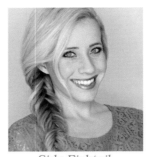

Side Fishtail,
page 58

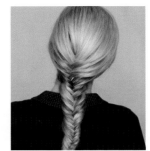

French Fishtail,
page 60

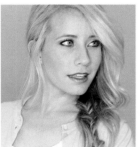

Red-Carpet Style,
page 62

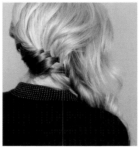

Elegance Swept to the
Side, page 64

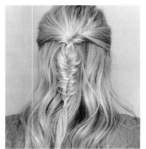

Half-Up Fishtail,
page 66

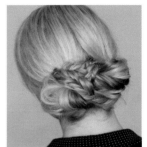

Fishtail Bun,
page 68

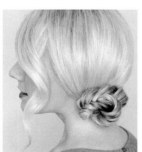

Fishtail Side Bun,
page 70

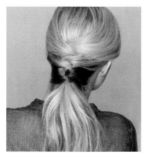

Crisscross
Ponytail, page 72

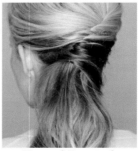

Formal Ponytail,
page 73

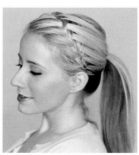

Waterfall Ponytail,
page 74

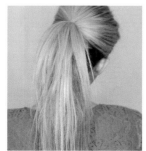

The Perfect Ponytail,
page 76

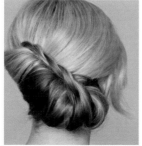

Twisted Chignon,
page 78

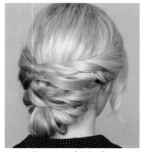

Twisted Updo,
page 80

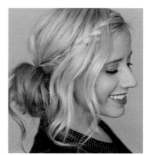

Waterfall Updo,
page 82

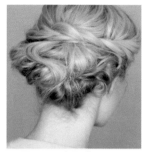

Twisted Bohemian Updo, page 84

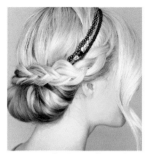

Simple Headband Updo, page 86

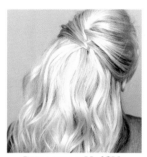

Crisscross Half-Up, page 88

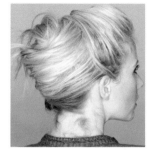

Crisscross French Twist, page 90

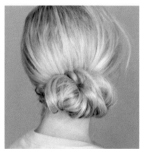

Fast Messy Bun, page 92

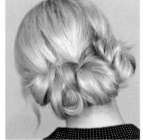

Three-Banded Buns, page 94

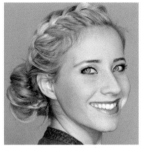

French Braided Messy Bun, page 96

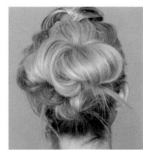

French Braided Pompadour, page 97

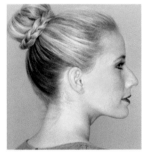

Braided Ballerina Bun, page 98

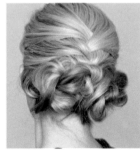

Rope Bun, page 100

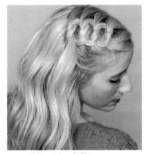

Knotted Bangs, page 102

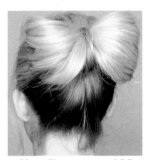

Hair Bow, page 103

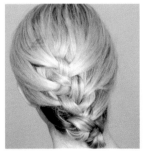

Knotty or Nice, page 104

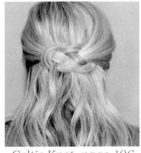

Celtic Knot, page 106

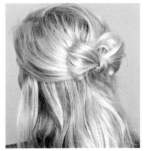

Half-Up Hair Bow, page 108

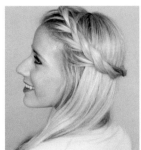

Twisted Halo, page 110

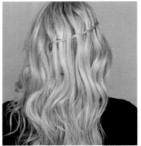

Waterfall Twist,
page 112

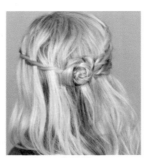

Waterfall Flower,
page 114

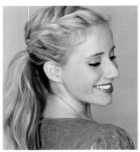

Bohemian Twist
Ponytail, page 116

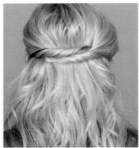

Twisted Together,
page 118

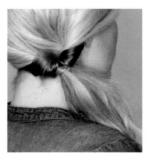

Simple Topsy
Tail, page 120

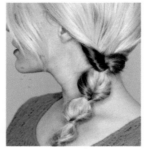

Topsy Tail Faux
Fishtail, page 121

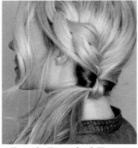

Dutch Braided Topsy
Tail, page 122

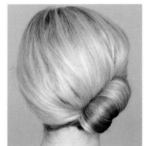

Topsy Tail Chignon,
page 124

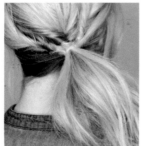

Layered Topsy Tail,
page 126

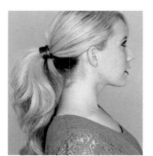

Wrapped Ponytail,
page 128

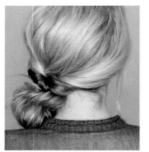

Topsy Tail Messy Bun,
page 130

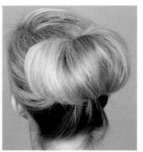

Topsy Tail
High Bun, page 131

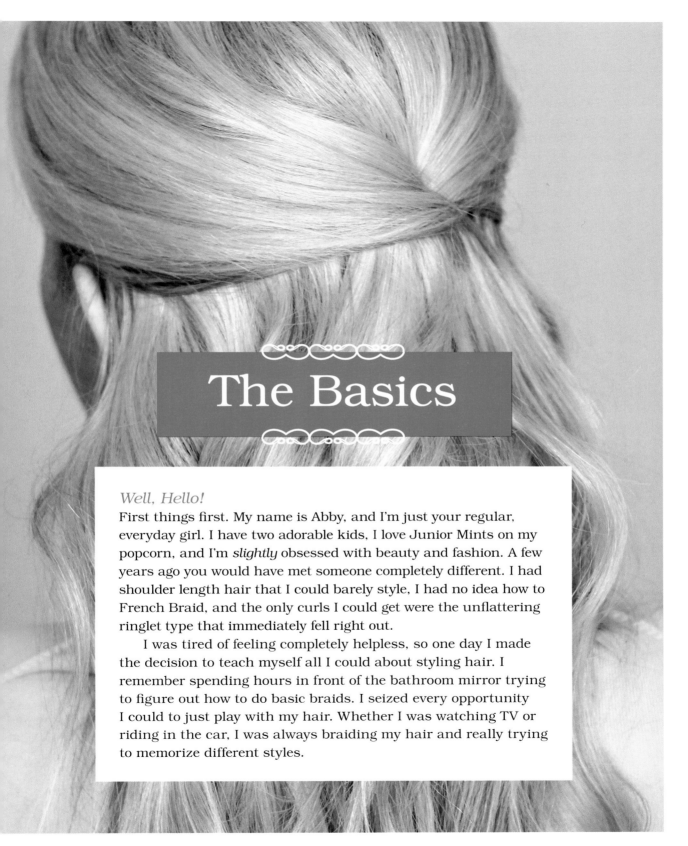

The Basics

Well, Hello!

First things first. My name is Abby, and I'm just your regular, everyday girl. I have two adorable kids, I love Junior Mints on my popcorn, and I'm *slightly* obsessed with beauty and fashion. A few years ago you would have met someone completely different. I had shoulder length hair that I could barely style, I had no idea how to French Braid, and the only curls I could get were the unflattering ringlet type that immediately fell right out.

I was tired of feeling completely helpless, so one day I made the decision to teach myself all I could about styling hair. I remember spending hours in front of the bathroom mirror trying to figure out how to do basic braids. I seized every opportunity I could to just play with my hair. Whether I was watching TV or riding in the car, I was always braiding my hair and really trying to memorize different styles.

This book is proof that if I could do it, so can you. I believe that styling hair isn't a talent. It's a skill. It's something that you learn and get better at through practice. I'm not a hairdresser, nor do I profess to be one. I'm just a girl with a passion for hair. I hope this book inspires you to learn and improve like I did, but most of all I hope it encourages you to discover a newfound confidence and a love for your hair and yourself.

As you learn these styles and start wearing them around, I promise you're going to feel like a million bucks. People are going to notice how beautiful you look, and it won't be because your hair looks fabulous—which, by the way, it will—but because you're walking a little taller and with an extra bounce in your step. So go on, learn a new hairstyle or two, because who knows? It just might change your life!

A Couple Things You Should Know about Me

I know what it's like to have miserable hair that refuses to grow. I had split ends for miles with no hope in sight for the long healthy hair I wanted. I started asking questions and talking to different stylists. They gave me invaluable advice, and I started buying new products and treating my hair differently. Within a couple years my hair went from hitting the tops of my shoulders to the middle of my back. It went from unhealthy and dull to lustrous, thick, and strong. It was absolutely beautiful and I babied it.

Over a year ago I hopped on the ombre train, but getting my blonde color back quickly become my worst nightmare. For months my hair was not only bright orange but just completely fried! Ahhhh! Can any of you relate? It's the worst feeling in the world to be completely embarrassed of your hair. Talk about a confidence killer! Like it or not, our hair is one of the most noticeable parts of our overall appearance. I wish it wasn't connected to how we feel about ourselves, but it is.

The point to my story is that if you don't have beautiful hair right now, it's something you can have. And it's something you should strive for! If you are patient, use the right products, and care for your hair the way you should, your hair will easily become your most favorite accessory.

So, Abby, how do I get this gorgeous hair you speak of?!

Oh, I'm so glad you asked!

Basic Hair Care

When to Wash

Let's talk about washing. How often are you washing your hair? If it's every day, I'm going to ask you to go to every other day. If you're washing it every other day, I'm going to ask you to go three days. I wash my hair maybe two times a week. I promise you'd never know! You want to minimize the amount of times you wash your hair, and here's why: The natural oils in your hair are hydrating and can benefit your hair more than any product. The problem with these oils is that they can also make our hair look, feel, and smell dirty. Lucky for us we can coax our scalp into producing less oil. It's all about supply and demand. The more you wash your hair and strip your hair of those natural oils, the more oil your scalp will produce. The less you wash your hair, the less oil your scalp will produce. You've got to train it. Don't go straight from washing every day to only once a week—that really will be gross! Gradually work up to it. In addition to healthier hair, you'll also have more time in the morning to try these gorgeous styles you're about to see!

Dry Shampoo

Invest in some dry shampoo. It looks like a can of hair spray but behaves completely differently. When sprayed on your roots, dry shampoo absorbs excess oil. It's a quick and easy way to get clean and fresh-smelling hair without washing. Dry shampoo will get you through one more day—or three more days if you're like me! Not only does dry shampoo freshen dirty hair, but it will also thicken your flyaways by weighing them down, and it will add texture and body to lifeless hair.

If you have fine or clean hair that you are trying to style, mist some dry shampoo all over and it will add texture and grip. This is great for creating the styles in this book, most of which were created with second-, third-, or fourth-day hair. Hey, don't judge! Working with clean hair can be hard to do—your hair just styles better when it's dirty. I didn't make the rules!

Shampoo and Conditioner

Okay, so far you know when to wash and what to do on the days in between. So when you finally do wash that dirty hair, does it matter what products you use? I'm going to go ahead and say yes on this one! If you're serious about having healthy hair, you don't have to spend an arm and a leg to get a quality shampoo and conditioner, but you do need to know your ingredients. You want a shampoo and conditioner that is sulfate- and paraben-free.

Sulfates are the ingredients in shampoo that cause it to lather. Lathering shampoo does the scrubbing for you. It strips your hair of all the products you've been using but all of your hair's natural oils, too. The price you pay for an easy wash is damaged hair. When you start using a sulfate-free shampoo, you're going to need to use a little elbow grease to clean your hair.

Massage your roots and gently detangle your hair with your fingers. Your hard work will definitely pay off.

If you color your hair, you want a shampoo and conditioner that also prevents your color from swirling down the drain. It makes no sense to spend a fortune on coloring your hair at a salon only to use hair-care products that strip the color at home. If you're blonde and need to brighten up or cool down the brassy golds, use a purple shampoo and/or conditioner. Using a purple product will breathe life back into your hair by distributing purple pigment that neutralizes the brassy, yellow tones. To see extensive, up-to-date reviews of my favorite products, be sure to visit my website, twistmepretty.com.

Split Ends

What causes them? How can you avoid them? Most split ends are caused by heat. One of the reasons I recommend washing only a couple times a week is because the more you wash your hair, the more you're forced to use heat. The blow-dryer, the straightener, the curling iron—the things that make our hair look the most gorgeous are also the things that cause the most damage. The heat from these tools weakens and destroys vital proteins in your hair as well as depletes your hair's natural oils. By washing your hair less, you're able to skip out on blowing it dry. And by learning new hairstyles, you're able to avoid straightening or curling it every day.

Other ways we get those nasty split ends include excessive combing and handling, poor diet, and—believe it or not—towel drying. Our hair is most vulnerable when wet, so take care when brushing and drying it. Instead of flipping your hair upside down and going to town on it with a towel, gently pat it dry or squeeze the water out of your hair.

Before subjecting your strands to high temperatures from irons and dryers, make sure to use a thermal-protecting serum, spray, mousse, or cream. Thermal products will not only shield your hair from the damaging effects of heat styling, but most products also have added UV inhibitors that prevent colors from fading and frizz caused by the harmful effects of the sun. Most thermal products will also strengthen and hydrate your hair while adding shine and gloss. Win-win!

Haircuts

How often should you be trimming your hair? I am not a hairdresser, so take my recommendations with a grain of salt. I would advise you to speak with your hair stylist about this and be very specific about your goals. I have been blessed to have some amazing hair stylists who took care of my hair, who offered me some of the best advice, and whom I trusted. With that said, I've also had a couple terrible stylists who ruined my hair. It's okay to doubt your stylist! Do your research and know what you want. Don't be afraid to talk and share your vision.

Knowing how often to cut your hair has a lot to do with your goals and the chemical processes you put your hair through on a regular basis. If your hair is long, to keep it looking healthy trim it every 12 to 15 weeks. Long hair is susceptible to breakage, and over time it can start looking stringy and thin. Getting regular trims will keep your long hair looking strong and healthy. For those with short or medium-length hair who are trying to grow it out, the same rules generally apply. Regular trims at 12-to-15-week intervals are important in keeping your hair healthy and split ends managed. If your stylist tells you to come in for a trim in 6 weeks . . . well, use your best judgment. If in 6 weeks your hair feels great, skip the trim and wait a little longer.

If you color, highlight, perm, or chemically straighten your hair on a regular basis, you may notice that your hair needs to be trimmed more frequently. If your hair is breaking or is very dry, more frequent haircuts may help prevent overdrying and further breakage. Remember, great stylists are there to help you and are more than happy to chat with you and offer advice. Don't be afraid to say what you want and what your long-term goals are.

Hair Types

There are basically four types of hair: straight, wavy, curly, and kinky. While knowing your natural hair type is very important, I feel it's even more important to know your strand texture and thickness. Before you begin any of these styles it's crucial you identify whether you have fine hair, coarse hair, or are somewhere in-between. Our goal is to work with our hair, not against it.

Fine Hair

If you have fine hair it means you have a small hair shaft. It doesn't necessarily mean your hair is thin, but sometimes that is the case. You have fine hair if your hair doesn't hold curl, breaks easily, is prone to flyaways, and usually hangs flat. While having fine hair can sometimes be hard to live with, you have the most room for dramatic transformation!

Fine-Hair Care

- Having oily hair is not uncommon for people with fine hair, and you may find you need to wash it more frequently than your coarse-haired friends. If you can afford to, though, skip a day or two, because like we talked about, washing can cause damage.

- Put conditioner on only the tips of your hair. By not conditioning the scalp, you can help keep your fine hair from looking limp.

- When wet, fine hair is very weak and prone to damage. Be extra gentle when you come out of the shower by not vigorously towel-drying, brushing, or styling your hair immediately as they could cause breakage.

- For maximum lift and volume, use mousse and a round brush at the roots when blowing hair dry.

- Use a hair-thickening shampoo and conditioner and also a thickening cream, serum, or spray. You can ask your stylist which product is right for you or head to your local beauty store for advice. Or a salon, but never a grocery store.

Fine-Hair Styling

Get a layered cut. You want to avoid your hair looking flat, and by adding in a few tapered layers it's going to create the illusion of fuller hair. The styles in this book will work with layered hair, but make sure any pieces that poke out look intentional. To get the styles looking their best, I recommend the following:

- Spray your hair with dry shampoo before you start styling. The dry shampoo will add texture and grip to your hair, making the pins and braids hold stronger. It will also add volume without matting or weighing down the hair.

- Tease your roots! Doing so will add much needed volume and texture. Take care and be gentle to avoid breakage.

- Use products that are light and do not weigh your hair down like heavy pomades and gels.

- If possible, work with wavy or curly hair. Having that added texture in your hair will add volume to all your styles. Avoid heat by sleeping in loose braids or using Velcro rollers.

- Set each hairstyle with Kenra Volume Spray 25—it's the best hair spray available.

Coarse Hair

If you have coarse hair, your strands are very thick. They're the mega strands! Your hair usually takes longer to dry than fine hair. It's most likely dry but it can tolerate heat and resist breakage.

Coarse-Hair Care

- Avoid washing your hair more than three times a week. Let those natural oils really soften up and moisturize the hair.

- Coarse hair can often look dull, but adding some shine serum to your routine should punch up the lustrousness of the hair.

- No lightweight products allowed. You need to reach for heavy-duty products such as firm-hold gels, hair sprays, and pomades.

- It's a good idea to give your coarse hair a weekly deep-conditioning treatment. This will ensure you keep the dryness under control.

- Before getting out of the shower, rinse your hair with cool water. This will cause the cuticles to close, which will seal in moisture and color.

Coarse-Hair Styling

- If your hair is frizzy and unmanage-able, invest in an anti-frizz serum. You can find fabulous serums that protect against heat, add shine, and eliminate frizz. By eliminating frizz, braids and twists will look smoother and more put together.

- If your hair is super thick, you will need to tease the roots and set with hair spray. Having coarse hair doesn't prevent you from having flat hair!

- Extra large bobby pins are a must. They hold more hair and are stronger, which will keep your braids and updos secure.

- Rather than using a million pins on one large section of hair, use fewer pins on smaller sections.

- If your hair is very thick, your updos and braids are going to look fuller than mine. Most times you'll be thankful for that! If it's annoying, though, pull your braids and twists extra tight.

Terminology and Tools

Common tools and accessories used throughout the book:
- duck-billed clips
- clips
- bobby pins (small and large)
- clear elastics
- 1-inch curling iron
- 1-inch straightener
- rattail comb
- Topsy Tail tool

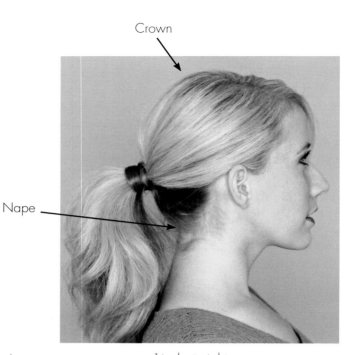

Crown

Nape

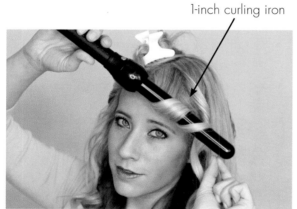

1-inch curling iron

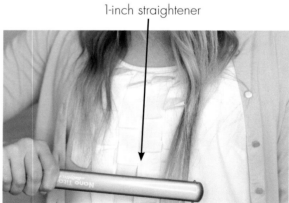

1-inch straightener

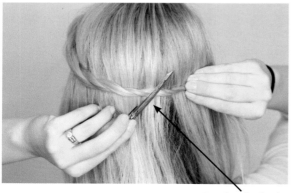

Duck-Billed Clip

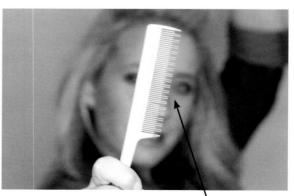

Rattail Comb

Basics Techniques

Teasing

Before I start every style I tease my hair. It makes a huge difference in the volume and also adds grip and texture to help hold some of the styles. It is so very important, please do not skip this first step! Any type of comb will do. I really like the classic rattail combs and also boar teasing combs. You can pick either up at most grocery and beauty supply stores.

1. Gather the section of hair you want teased. I usually start from the back and work my way around to the front. Take your comb and place it 4 or 5 inches away from your scalp. Then you're going to pull the comb down toward your scalp, creating a whole bunch of knots and snarls.

2. Next spray your snarls with your favorite hair-spray. Mine is the Kenra 25 super-hold finishing spray.

3. Take your comb and softly brush out some of the noticeable snarls. Make sure you don't brush out all the snarls you've just created, just the ones on top peeking through.

4. Work your way around to the front. Keep combing through those noticeable snarls.

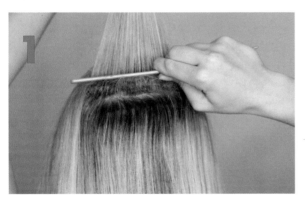
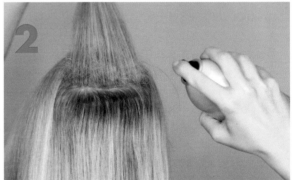
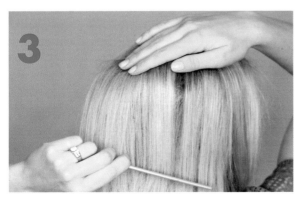
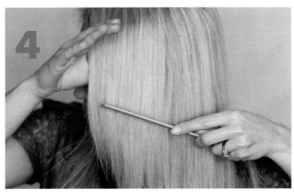

There is a very fine line between teasing just enough and teasing too much. The goal is to add a little bit of volume and texture. You want to maintain your head shape, and you want it to look natural. You definitely do not want snarls peeking through. Even if you end up brushing out most of the snarls, roughing up and spraying those strands will really make a difference!

Blow-Drying

There are many different ways to blow-dry your hair, and this is simply what works for me. I don't like to flip my head upside down because I find I get more flyaways near my part when I do. Before you begin blow-drying, towel dry your hair, comb through it, and apply your product or root lift if needed.

1. Start by blowing out your bangs. If you swoop your bangs, dry them the opposite way they lie and it will ensure you get the perfect swoop.

2. Once your bangs are completely dry, go onto drying the rest of your roots.

3. Next take a paddle brush or round brush, whichever you prefer, and brush out the rest of your hair as you blow it dry.

Getting a good blow out is very important. Do your best to get your hair as smooth as possible while you're blowing it dry. You want to avoid any touch-up's with the straightener as that direct heat is much harsher on your hair.

Pancaking

This is a term I will use often, and it basically means to spread out and flatten a braid. Doing this will make your braid look fuller and add great texture.

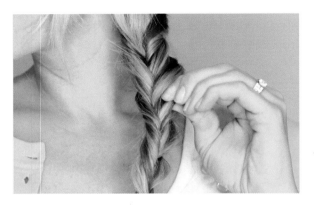

Creating a Simple Half-Up and Sliding in a Bobby Pin

This technique is used throughout the book. You're basically folding the hair over itself and pinning the outside pieces of hair. I started this style by curling my hair with a 1-inch wand. See pages 22–23.

1. Start by teasing your roots and combing through the snarls. Using your index fingers, loosely pull back the top layers of hair. You only want the very top layers; if you pull all the thickness back, the bobby pins will not hold.

2–5. You are basically going to fold the hair over itself. Combine the hair into your dominant hand, and with your non-dominant hand start folding the hair over.

6. Holding the hair in place with your non-dominant hand, open up your bobby pin with the flat side on top and slide it into the seam. You only need to pin those very outer layers on the fold because they're the ones holding the style in place.

Tips

If one bobby pin doesn't hold the style, go ahead and use a couple more. I like to bring a little bit more hair over from the side and add it to the fold before I pin. If the pins aren't holding the style, make sure you're using sturdy bobby pins and you're not asking the pins to hold too much! You're just pinning those very top layers of hair.

Be sure to buy high-quality bobby pins. They make a huge difference! I buy my bobby pins from Sally Beauty Supply, and they are super strong. I've never had a bobby pin fold in on me, and they grip the hair better than the cheap ones. So before you get frustrated with yourself for not being able to slide in a bobby pin, make sure you've got the right bobby pins for the job!

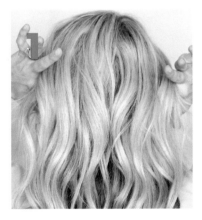
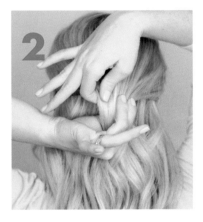
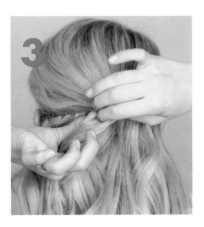
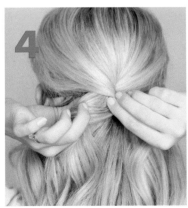
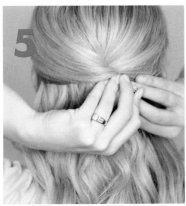
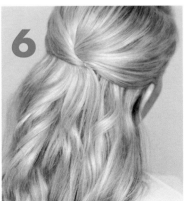

Basic Pompadour

This is a great style to choose when you've let your hair air-dry or when it's lacking volume. It really lifts your eyes up and makes you look more alert. I started this style with left over 1-inch wand curls (see pages 22–23).

1. Using the outside arch of the eyebrows as a guide, section off the top layers of hair. Make sure not to take the full section of hair, just those very top layers.

2. I like to tease my hair with a good old-fashioned rattail comb.

3. Take a comb and tease the roots by pulling the comb toward the scalp. Run your fingers through the hair making sure no snarls are visible but taking care not to brush out all the volume.

4. You're going to loosely pull that section of hair back and twist the hair where you want to secure it. Slide a bobby pin or two into the twist. If you find it easier, you may slide in two bobby pins, making sure to crisscross them at the center. Then take a comb and tease the sides and back of the hair to add in a little bit more volume.

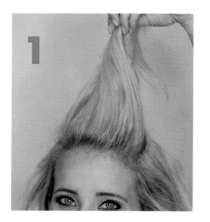

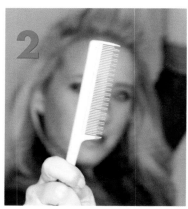

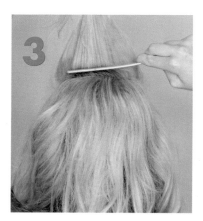

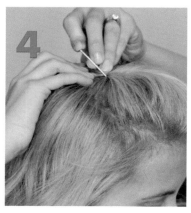

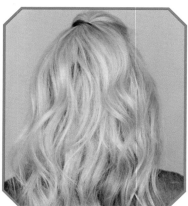

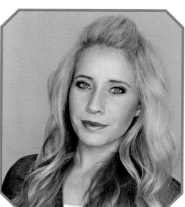

Beach Waves

1. Section off top layers of hair using any type of clips.

2. Split the bottom layer into a few sections. Take one of the sections and twist it away from your face using your index finger. Run your straightener over the twist. As you clamp the iron on the twist, the hair should flatten out a bit. The tighter your twist, the tighter your waves. If you want looser waves like mine, allow the straightener to really flatten out that twist.

3. Using a duck-billed clip, attach the twist to the hair near your scalp.

4. Continue taking sections and warming up the twists. Once you've twisted all your hair, let the twists set. The longer you leave them in, the longer your waves are going to stay. I'd recommend at least ten minutes. Finish putting on your makeup and go do some dishes.

5. Release the twists.

6. Gently run your fingers through the twists.

7 Continue until the twists are loose but not totally gone.

Tip

A beach spray is the perfect finishing touch for this hairstyle. It will add more texture, boost the waves, and add body and volume to your hair. The texture is what's so amazing about this style. This is the perfect texture for a great messy bun and also to have before you start any type of braid.

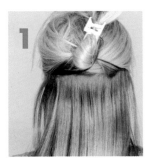
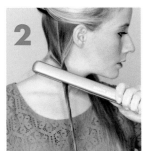
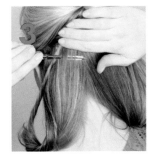
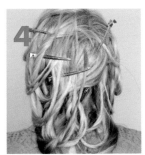
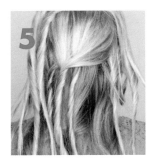
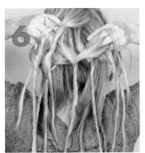
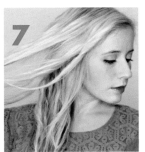
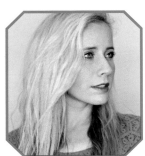

Wand Curls

This is one of the easiest ways to curl your hair. You literally cannot mess it up! I can get through my entire head of hair in less than ten minutes. You will need a 1-inch curling iron and a good heat serum.

1. Section off your hair from the ears on up. Spray the hair that's down with a heat serum.

2. Take 1- to 2-inch sections, depending on the texture of your hair, and wrap the section away from your face around the curling iron. Keep a hold on the end of the hair. You don't want that wrapped around the iron.

3. Continue wrapping and curling each section.

4. You may alternate the direction of your curls, but when it comes to anything near your face, always wrap away.

5. Release a section of hair from what you have clipped up and continue to curl.

6. Remember to wrap anything near your face away.

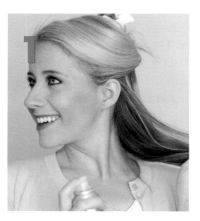
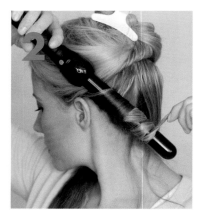
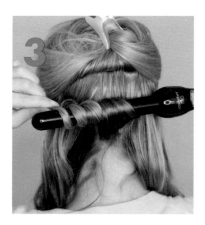
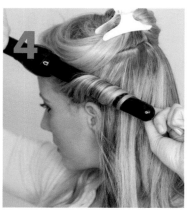
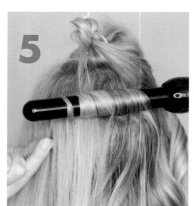
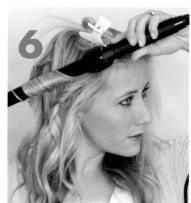

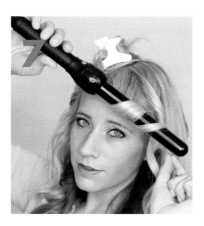
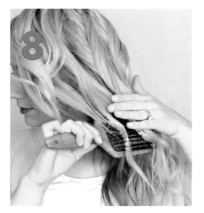
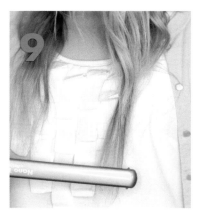

7. When you get to the bangs, use your 1-inch or larger barreled iron to create a looser curl in the front. My iron is 1-¼ inches in diameter.

8. Gently brush out the curls to loosen them.

9. Straightening the ends is really important when it comes to the way your curls lay. Feel free to leave the ends of your hair out of the curling process, but if you have frizzy ends you'll probably need to straighten them.

Tip

If you want looser curls, you don't need to head straight for the larger barreled curling iron. Try taking a paddle brush and passing it through the curls to loosen them up. These curls are gorgeous on days three and four, because as they loosen up you're left with a really pretty wave that doesn't fall out.

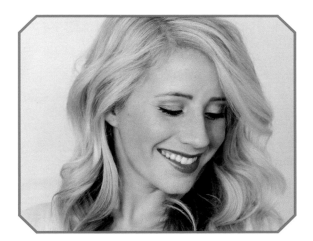

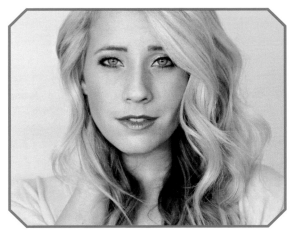

Straightener Curls

Here is the simplest way to get great curls using a straightener.

1. Section off the hair from your ears up.

2. Bring a small section forward from behind the ears. You're going to start with your knuckles facing down, or away from you, on the flat iron. Clamp the hair at the roots.

3. Slowly rotate your wrist so that your knuckles are up, or close to your face, all while pulling the straightener down the hair shaft. It's all in the wrist!

4. Repeat those steps taking small sections from each layer and clamping the straightener down near the roots. Remember to start with your knuckles facing down, away from you. Then rotate your wrist so that your knuckles are now close to your face and begin pulling down the hair.

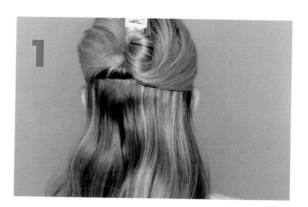

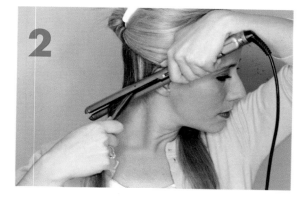

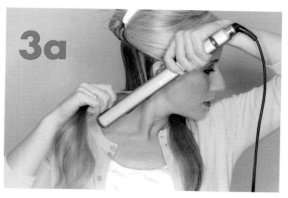

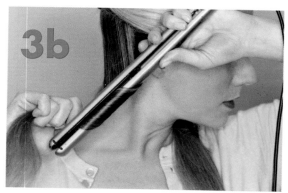

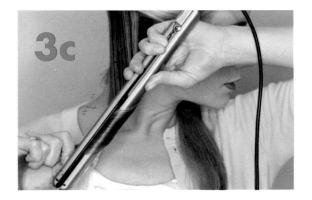

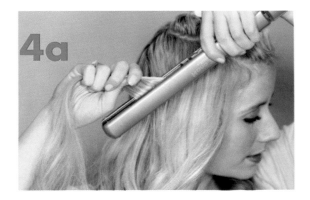

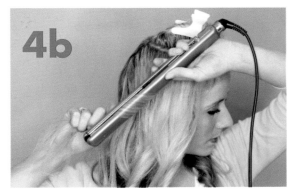

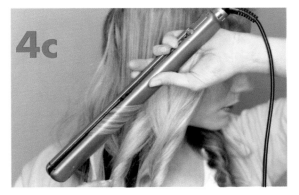

Tip

I like to split my hair into three layers, one right at the ears, one at my temples, and one small section up top. From each layer, I curl three to four sections of hair. To finish, I finger through the curls to separate any that are stuck together. Then I tease the roots and spray with either a texturizing spray and/or a hair spray.

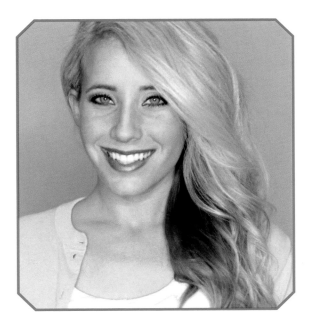

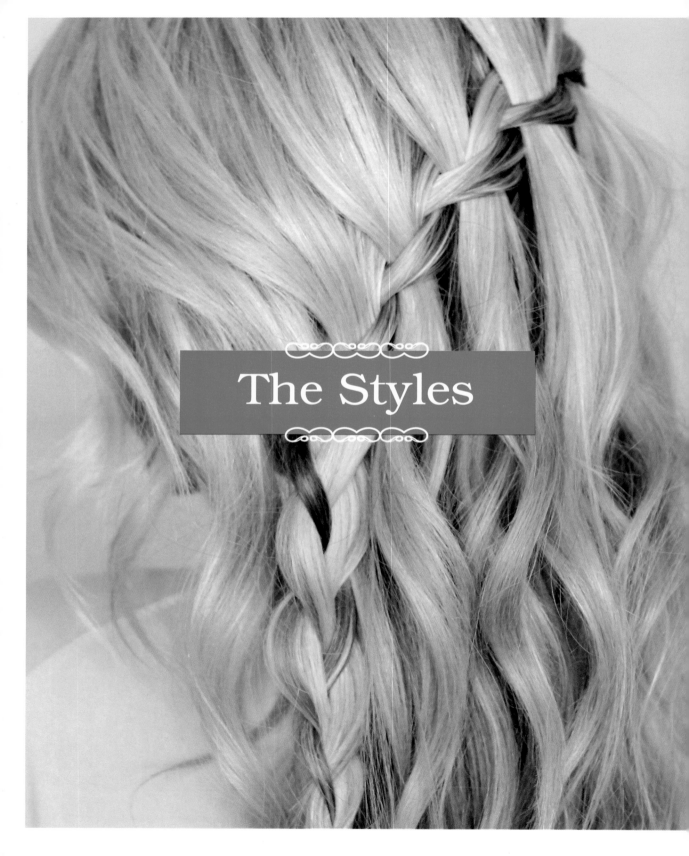

The Styles

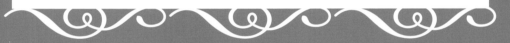

Braids

The hairstyles in this section are ones you absolutely need to learn before moving on to more advanced styles. They are your foundational braids and twists. Skipping these styles would be like moving onto algebra before you know your times tables—you just wouldn't do it! If you can learn these basic styles, the rest of this book will be a piece of cake. I suggest at first you don't watch yourself in the mirror. Instead, practice while looking at my step-by-steps. Once you think you have it down, show me! I'd love to see you master these basics and all the styles in this book. Tag photos of your braids to @twistmepretty on Instagram.

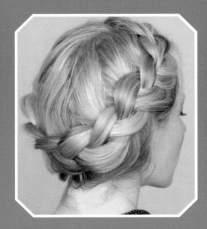
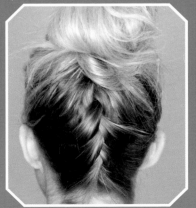
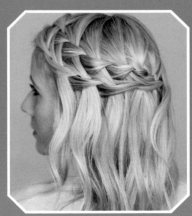

Basic French Braid

Remember: you are braiding, adding a section of hair to one of the outermost strands, braiding, adding a section of hair to the outermost strand on the other side, braiding, etc. Move super slow, and don't let all the words confuse you.

1. Separate the hair into three sections. Hold the left section in the left hand, the right section in the right hand, and the middle section in between your right hand's index finger and thumb. The placement is very important.

2. Using your left hand, place the left section OVER the middle section and grab it with your right hand.

3. Hold the new left section in your left hand and the new middle section in between your right hand's index finger and thumb. With your left hand, reach over the middle section and pull the right section OVER the middle section. Basically you just started a three-strand braid, nothing too fancy.

4. Now you're going to start incorporating the rest of the hair into the braid. Place all three sections in your right hand. The left section should be held by your index finger and thumb. Using your left index finger, pull a section of hair that is the same thickness as the other sections from the front left and incorporate it into that left section.

5. Pull this section in at a slight angle.

6. Now you're going to do another regular braid. Start by bringing the left section, the one you just added hair to, OVER the middle section with your left hand. Grab it with your right hand's index finger and thumb.

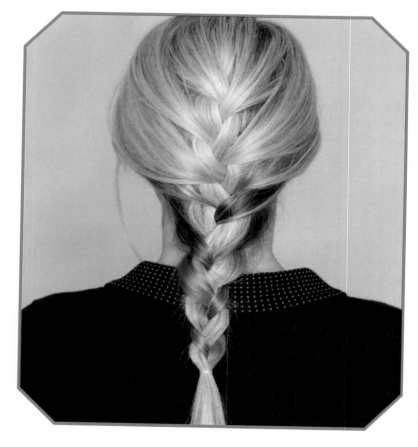

7. Move all three strands into your left hand and repeat. With your right hand, add a new section of hair to the right strand, bring it OVER the middle piece, and grab it with your left hand.

8–9. Repeat until you have a perfect French Braid.

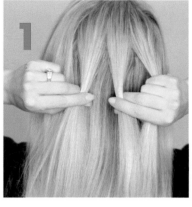

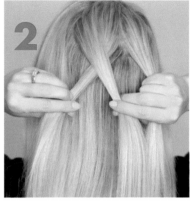

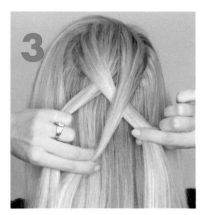

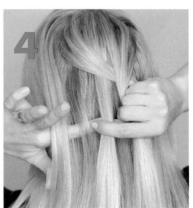

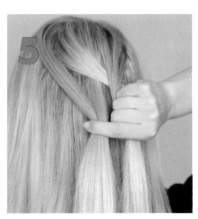

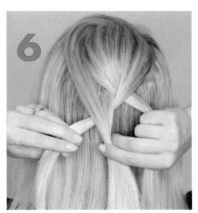

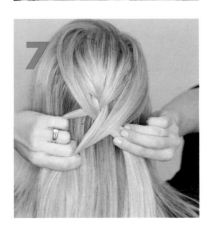

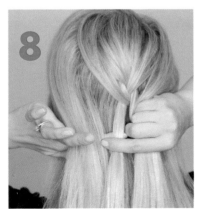

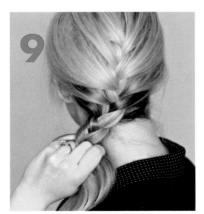

Rope Braid

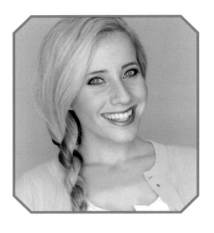

1–2. Gather all the hair to one side. Split the hair into two equal sections and start by twisting them in the same direction. It doesn't matter which direction, but they must be twisting the same way. I am twisting mine toward my face.

3–4. To create the rope braid, twist the two sections together in the opposite direction. I am twisting mine away from my face because I twisted the individual sections toward my face.

5. Once you reach the end, tie off the braid with a clear elastic. Pancake these pieces by spreading the twists.

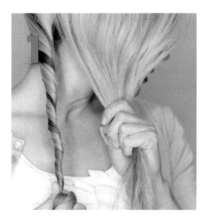

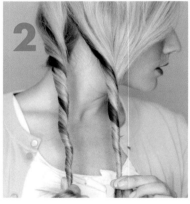

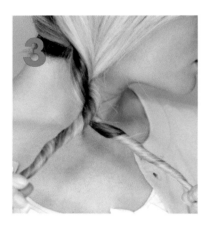

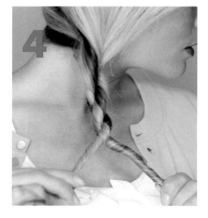

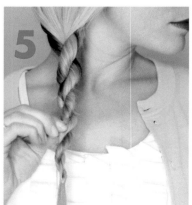

Tip

If you want more volume, tease the sections before you begin twisting.

Alternative Braid

Out of all the hairstyles in this book, the Alternative Braid is hands down my go-to. When I'm finished with the style I like to take the end of my rattail comb and slide it in near my temples. Then I gently pull up on the comb to give my roots just a bit more volume.

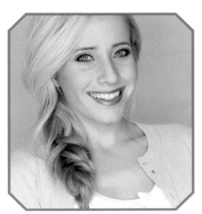

1. Tease your roots, gather all the hair to one side, and split the hair into two sections.

2. Using your index fingers, twist the sections toward each other.

3. Combine the twists with your non-dominant hand.

4. Put your free index finger through the twists.

5. Split the hair into two new sections.

6. Twist the section toward each other and repeat.

7. Pancake the braid by pull and tugging on those sections. Doing this will turn the average braid into one people really notice. Tie off with a clear elastic band and spray with your favorite hair spray.

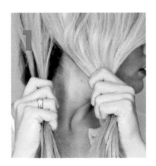
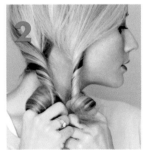
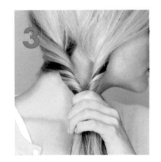
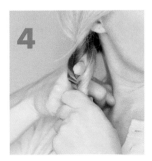
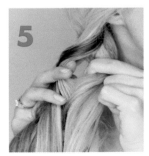
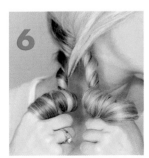
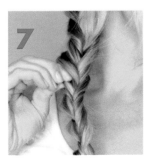

Falling Bohemian Twist

Basic Steps: divide hair into two sections, twist up, add more hair to each section, twist up, repeat. I started this style with left over 1-inch wand curls.

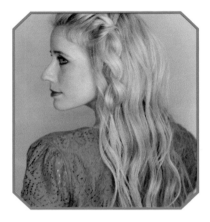

1. Take a triangular section of hair near the part and divide into two sections.

2. Take the bottom section and twist over the top section, or twist up.

3. Place both sections in your top hand, holding the bottom section with your index finger and thumb. With your free index finger, add a new section of hair to the bottom section, the one being held by your index finger and thumb.

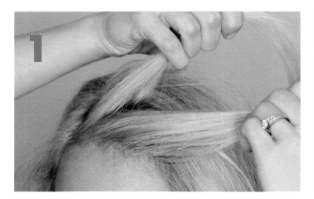

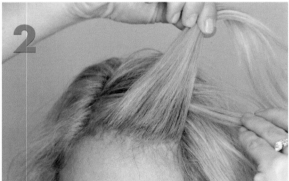

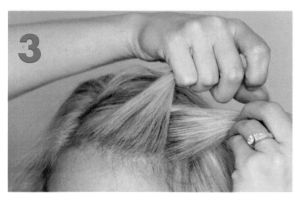

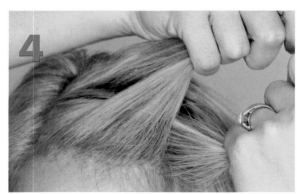

4. Transfer the sections into your bottom hand, holding the top section with your index finger and thumb. With your free index finger, add a new section of hair to the top section.

5. Twist the bottom section over the top section and repeat.

6. Continue adding and twisting until you reach your temple. From here, stop adding in new sections and just twist the remainder of hair.

7. Once you reach the bottom of the sections, tie them off with a clear elastic band. Hold the elastic with your index finger and thumb, knuckles directed away from you. Then turn your wrist toward your face to tighten the twist.

8. Take your other hand and hold that last section of hair you added in before starting your regular twist, release the elastic and insert a bobby pin to hold the style tight and in place.

Tip

After you've pinned the last section in place, the bottom twist is going to unravel a bit. I like to pancake the twist even more, especially up near my part. The fuller the twist, in my opinion, the more beautiful.

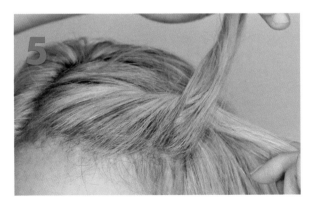

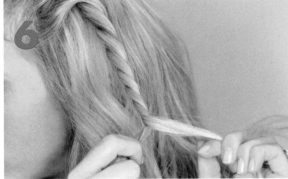

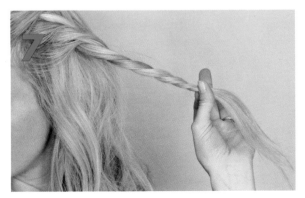

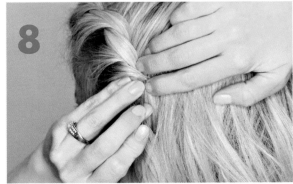

Bohemian Crown

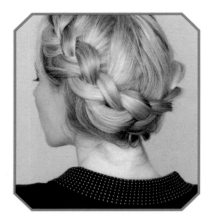

1. Begin a basic Dutch French Braid (see page 48). The outer sections are going UNDER the middle section.

2. Keep braiding, staying close to your hairline.

3. Keep the braid tight; you can always loosen it later.

4. At the nape of your neck, change direction. Hold all sections in your bottom hand . . .

5. . . . bring your top hand around your face and start braiding up. It may feel a little backward and you might lose the rhythm of the braid. Do not let go of the sections! Remember the steps and repeat them out loud. If my fingers ever get confused, I just start telling myself what to do out loud and it really helps.

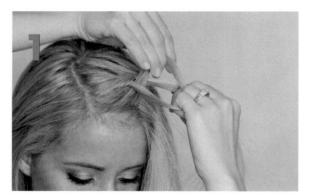

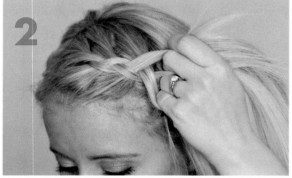

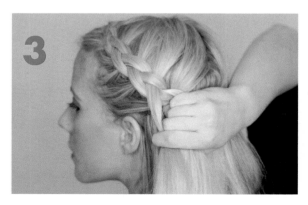

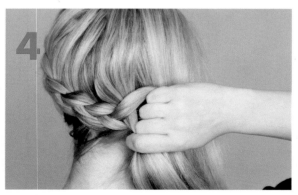

6. Keep the braid tight and close to your hairline.

7. When you've added in all the hair, continue a regular braid until you run out of hair.

8. Tie off with a clear elastic band.

9. Pin underneath your Dutch Braid where your braid ended.

10. And my favorite part, pancake the braid. Pull on the strands and make them as big and fluffy as your layers will allow. This is what makes the style look so pretty!

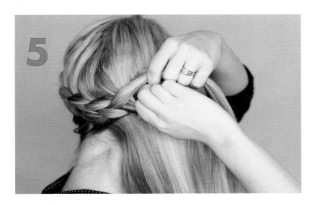

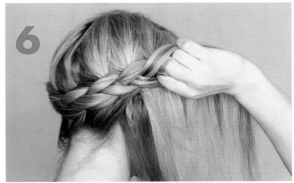

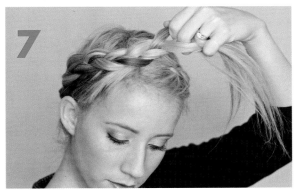

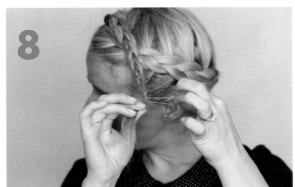

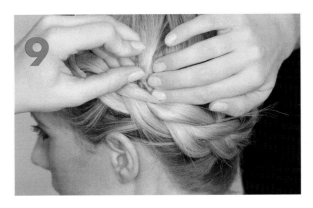

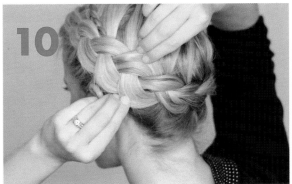

Braided Crown

Start this style out by curling the hair with a 1-inch wand and teasing the roots.

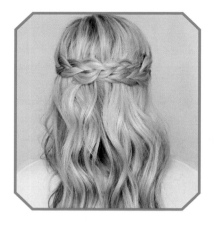

1. Gather a small section of hair, and divide the hair into three sections.

2. Braid these sections of hair.

3. While holding the end of the braid with one hand, flatten out the braid. Tug and pull up on the braid to make it look bigger and fuller.

4. Tie off the braid.

5. Repeat on the other side.

6. Loosely drape one of the braids across the back of your head and secure with bobby pins. You may need to roll the ends of your hair and secure them discretely with another pin.

7. Take the other braid and drape it directly over the pins and the first braid.

8. Secure with bobby pins.

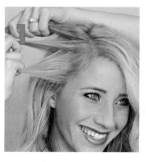
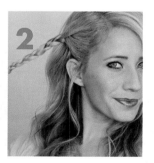
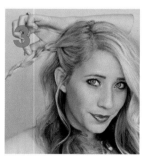
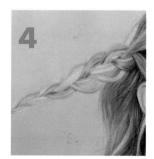
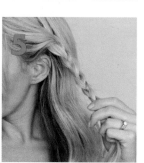
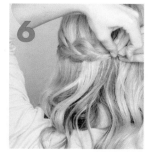
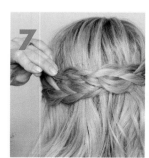
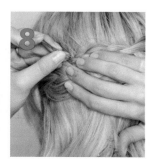

Braided Ponytail

Follow the steps 1–6 on the Braided Crown hairstyle.

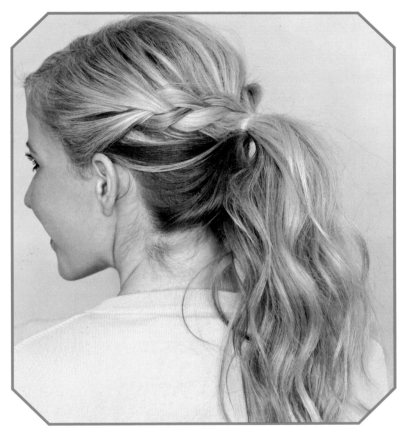

Tip

To finish off this look tease the ponytail and spray it with some texturizing beach spray.

1. Tie the braids together using a clear elastic band.

2. Remove the clear elastic bands holding the braids secure.

3. Use another clear elastic band to tie the rest of the hair up into a ponytail.

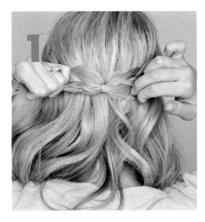

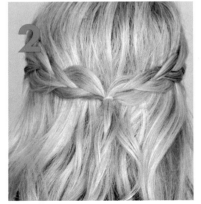

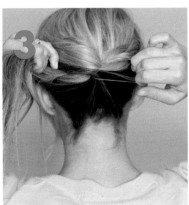

Chinese Staircase Stitch

I was obsessed with boondoggle as a kid. Do you remember the stuff? I spent hours making key chains and bracelets and trading them with my friends. Turns out boondoggle uses the Chinese Staircase Stitch. It's a really fun and easy knot that also works in your hair!

1. Gather the hair to one side. This is going to be the center section.

2. Take a small section of hair from the back of the center section.

3. Bring it over the center section making sure to leave a nice hole. It's going to resemble the number four.

4. Reach through the hole with the hand that is closest to the hole and grab the end of that strand.

5. Pull it through and combine it back into the center section. Congrats, you've just created one side of your Chinese Staircase Braid! Continue by just braiding down like I've done, or you can do a regular Chinese Staircase Stitch by bringing the next section the opposite way.

6. When you get to the end, tie it off with a clear elastic band.

7. To make it more interesting, I've gone ahead and braided my bangs back!

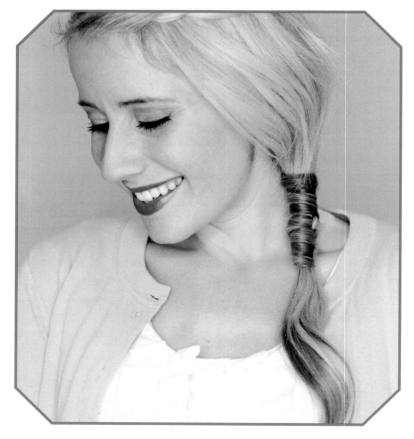

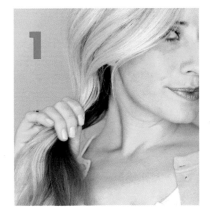

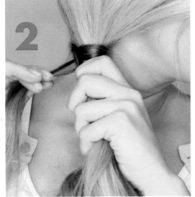

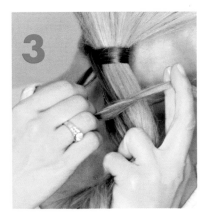

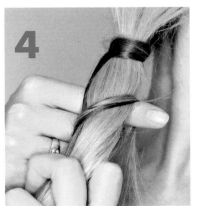

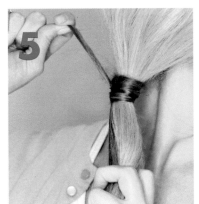

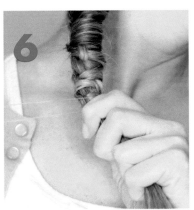

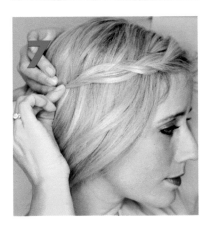

Play Around!

The Chinese Staircase Stitch I'm wearing is one-sided and the detail is all in the back. You can also play around with where you knot the hair. If you want the detail in the front, sweep the new section of hair away from your face instead of toward it. For a fun effect you can twirl your one-sided stitch around so it looks more like a spiral staircase. Play around with this style because it's a fun one!

French Braided Topknot

Braiding upside down is always a little bit tricky. It took me good while to really nail it. I suggest going very slow and saying the steps out loud. It'll help you remember what you're doing and what step you're on while calming down those confused little fingers! *You can do it. Practice, practice, practice!!*

1. Pull half the hair up in a high topknot. I used the Fast Messy Bun on pages 92–93.

2. Flip the hair upside down. If you have a ton of flyaways, now would be a good time to give them a good spray. Gather a small section of hair at the nape of your neck and split it into three sections.

3-5. French Braid the hair all the way up. Periodically look in the mirror to make sure those last chunks of hair added into the French Braid match the angle of the hair that's half up. You don't want to have to redo the braid because there's a large gap or unwanted bubbles.

6. When you get to the end, tie off with a clear elastic band and tie the remaining ends into another messy bun. The braid is tied off separately in case your Messy Bun doesn't have the shape you want. This way you can pull it out and redo it until you get the perfect one. You know how Messy Buns are!

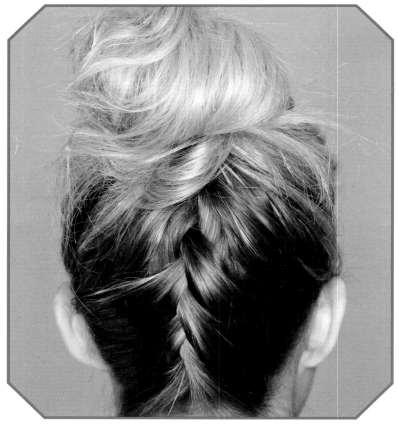

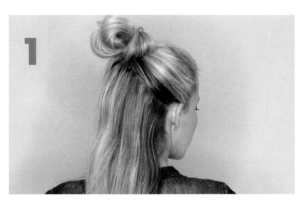

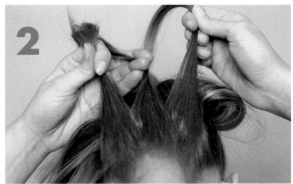

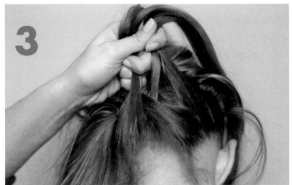

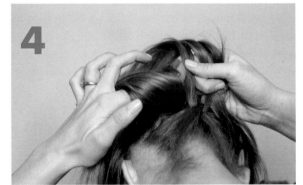

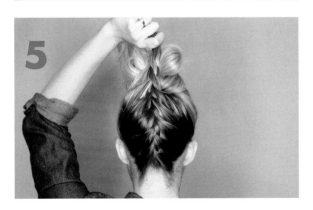

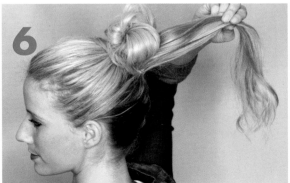

Waterfall Braid

Basic steps: Braid, transfer left and middle sections into your top hand, and drop the bottom piece. Replace the bottom piece with a new section. Braid the new bottom piece over the middle and repeat.

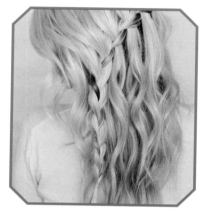

3. Next to the section you just dropped and right under the two sections you're holding in your top hand, gather a brand new section to braid with. Look at my bottom hand, that is a brand new section. We simply dropped the original and are gathering a new bottom section to use.

4. Gather all three sections in your top hand, braid the new bottom section over the middle, and then transfer all three sections into your bottom hand with the top section in between your index finger and thumb.

5. Start adding in new hair up top like you would a regular French Braid. Add hair to that top section. Braid it over the middle and transfer the left and middle sections into your top hand.

6. Drop that bottom piece.

7. Add in a new section of hair to replace the dropped bottom piece.

8. Repeat steps 5–7.

9. Once you've wrapped the braid around your crown, you can either secure it by sliding in a bobby pin or braiding it down and securing it with a clear elastic band.

1. Start with a simple three-strand braid near your part: bottom section over middle and top section over middle.

2. Transfer the top and middle sections into your top hand and let that bottom section fall.

Tips

The Waterfall Braid is one of my favorite hairstyles. It's gorgeous enough for prom but can easily be dressed down to wear to the gym. Technically this style isn't a basic braid because it's building off the French Braid. However, it's used in so many different styles throughout the book that I wanted to show you how to do it up front.

Before you begin you'll need to be proficient at French Braiding. If you're still learning your basic French Braid, this style is just going to frustrate you. But if the French Braid comes naturally to you, you'll be pleasantly surprised how easy it is!

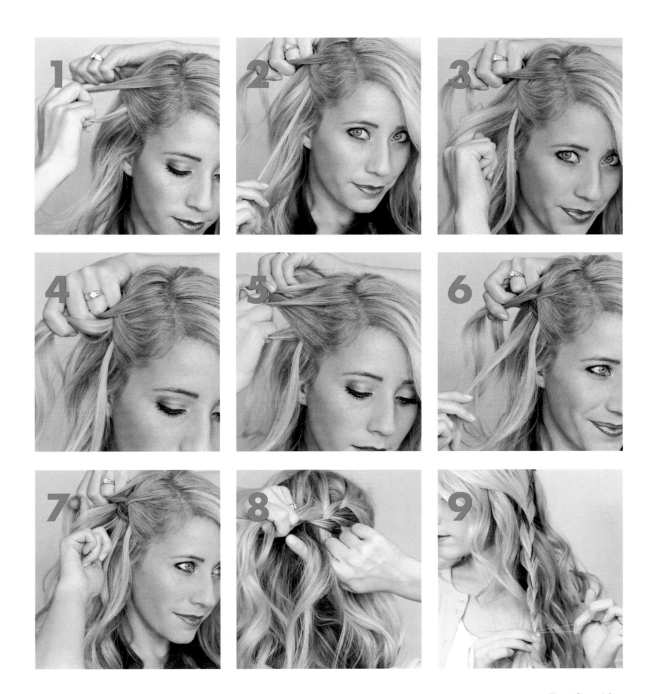

ᙏᙙDoubleᙙBraidsᙙᙘ

Start this hairstyle with leftover 1-inch wand curls. The basic steps are to make a Waterfall Braid on the top section of hair. Then make another Waterfall Braid directly underneath. Secure with bobby pins.

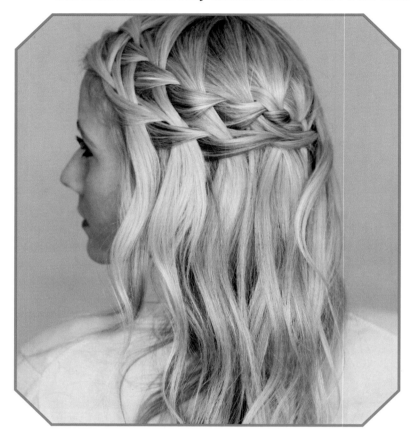

 Remove the duckbill clip and using the technique behind the Simple Half-Up hairstyle (see pages 18–19), fold those very outer layers over and secure them by sliding in a bobby pin or two.

Tip

Quick refresher on the Waterfall Braid: Braid the top section over the middle, then the bottom section over middle. Transfer top and middle sections into your top hand and drop that bottom piece. Replace the bottom piece with a new section. Braid the new bottom piece over the middle and repeat. Another way to style Double Braids is to pull the rest of the hair up into a ponytail. It adds a lot of texture and interest and is always fun to wear on race or game day!

1. An inch or so from the front of your hairline, begin a Waterfall Braid.

2. Drop the bottom piece.

3. Add in new hair and continue braiding.

4. Once you waterfall back and around as far as you'd like to go, finish by doing a three-strand braid with the ends. Secure with a duckbill clip.

5. Start another Waterfall Braid directly below the first one.

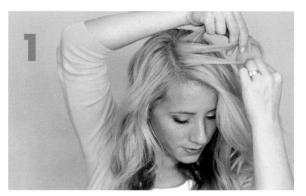

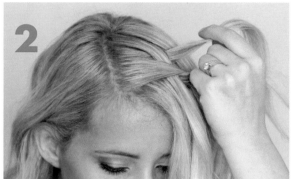

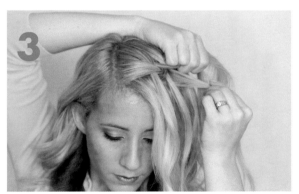

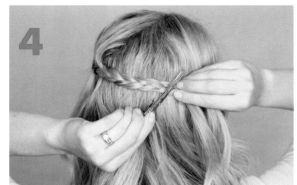

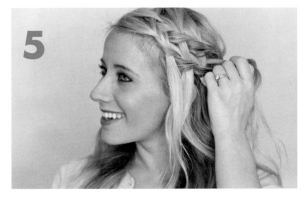

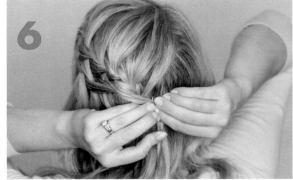

Milkmaid Braids

This is a great way to style your hair when it's getting a bit dirty and you can't save any of the curls or texture.

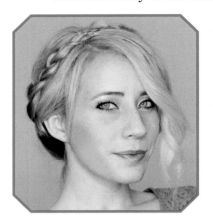

1. Divide the hair into two sections and braid each with just your basic braided piggies.

2. After securing with a clear elastic band, spread the braids.

3. Pull one of the braids up and over the top of your head, securing it with bobby pins. Repeat on the other side.

4. If there is a bubble near your ear from where the braid began, just tuck it in place with a bobby pin. Repeat on the other side.

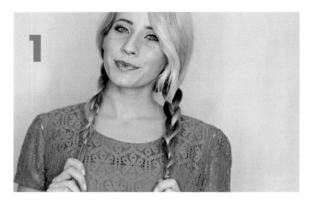

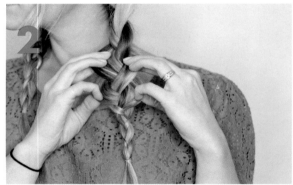

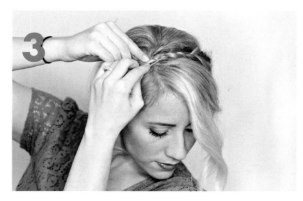

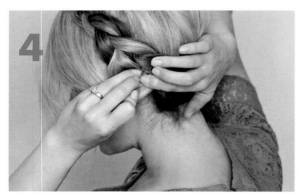

Dutch Braids

The Dutch Braid is a beautifully defined braid that sits on top of the hair. It's also known as an Inverted Braid or an Inside-Out French Braid. A Dutch Braid and a French Braid are one and the same, except with the Dutch Braid you braid the sections under the middle instead of over. One of my favorite things to do with a Dutch Braid is to pancake it. By spreading the sections, it makes the braid look so full and defined. The shape of a Dutch Braid is just gorgeous, so have fun learning these styles, because they're some of my favorites!

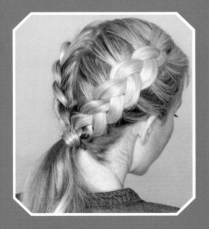 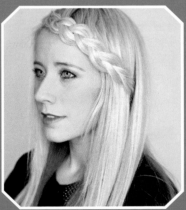 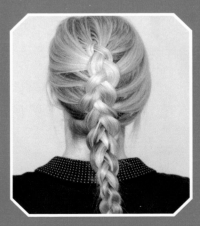

Dutch French Braid

If you mastered the French Braid this hairstyle will be a cinch!

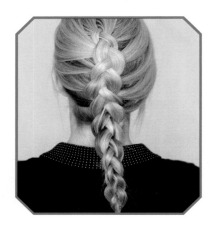

1. Separate the hair into three sections. Hold the left section in the left hand, the right section in the right hand and the middle section in between your right hands index finger and thumb.

2. Using your left hand, place the left section UNDER the middle section and grab with your right hands index finger and thumb. You'll need to hold that left piece in your hand and not in your index finger and thumb like in the picture. I just wanted to make sure you could clearly see the three strands.

3. With your left index finger and thumb, reach under the middle section and pull the right section UNDER the middle section.

4. Now you're going to start incorporating the rest of the hair into the braid. Place all three sections in your right hand. The left section in your index finger and thumb.

5. Using your left index finger, grab a new piece of hair from the front that is the same thickness as the existing sections and add it into the left section, the one that your right hand's index finger and thumb are holding.

6. Next, you're going to braid the left section, the one you just added hair into, UNDER the middle section. Grab it with your right hand's index finger and thumb. In the photo, I am holding that right section away from the other three so you can see the individual sections. Normally it is held in my ring finger and pinky so that my index finger and thumb are free to grab the new section.

7. Move all three sections into your left hand and repeat by using your index finger from your right hand to grab a piece of hair from the front and incorporate it into the right strand. Then bring it UNDER the middle section. Repeat until you have a gorgeous Dutch French Braid.

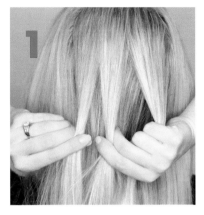
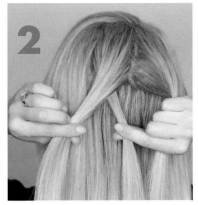
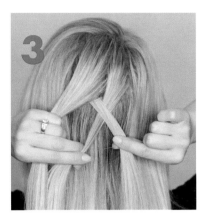
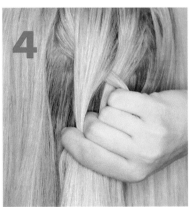
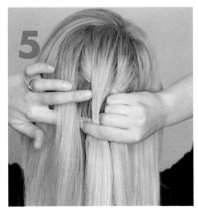
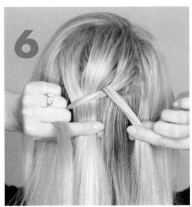
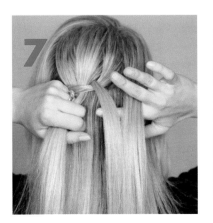

 Tip

This technique is exactly the same as the French Braid except you are braiding the pieces UNDER the middle section instead of over. Again these steps are a little wordy but the basic technique applies: braid left under middle, right under middle. Add hair to one of the sides, braid under the middle, add hair to the other side, braid under the middle, and so on.

ꙮLace Braidꙮ

Basic Steps: Make a one-sided Dutch French Braid (see pages 48–49) and wrap it around to above your ear. Tie it off with clear elastic band and secure the braid to your head with a bobby pin.

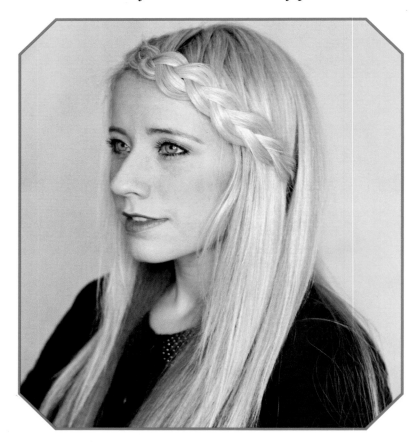

1. Start with a deep part. Gather a section of hair from the back of your part and divide it into three sections.

2. Begin a Dutch French Braid. Keep the braid tight and angle it forward, toward your face. Notice that the Dutch French Braid is only an inch or so thick.

3-4. Once you reach your forehead, you're going to begin a one-sided Dutch French Braid. This means you are only adding a new section of hair to the top strand, never to the strand closest to your face, and you are braiding UNDER the middle section. If this throws off your rhythm, just pretend you're adding in a new section like you normally would until it just comes naturally to you. I like to just twist my wrist. Look at it carefully in this picture and compare it to the next.

5. Gather a new section of hair from the back, where your Dutch French Braid started, and add to that top strand.

6. Now that you've combined that new section with the top strand, you're going to braid it under the middle.

7. Take that bottom strand, the one closest to your face and immediately braid it under the middle strand without adding any new sections of hair. It's easiest to just twist your wrist.

8. Once you get to about your temples start a regular braid. When you get to the bottom clip it off and pancake the sections to make the braid look fuller and more voluminous.

9. Tie the braid off with a clear elastic band and secure it underneath the top layers by crisscrossing bobby pins.

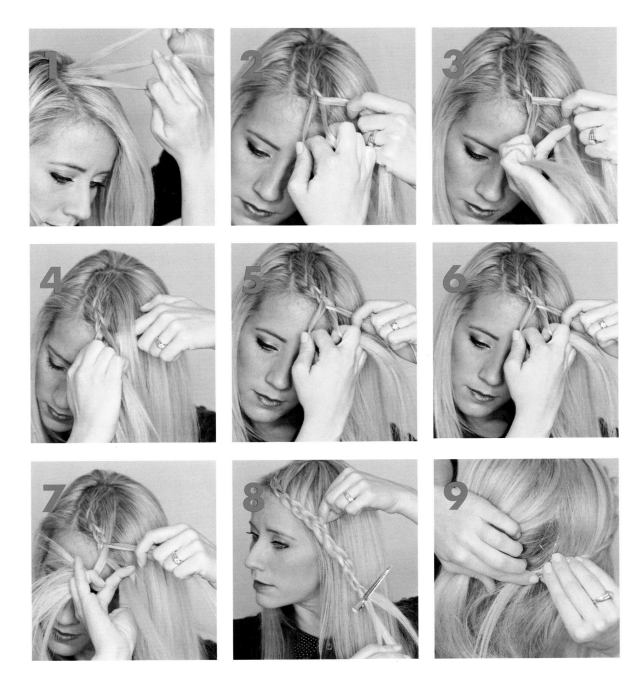

Dutch Braided Headband

I love this hairstyle because the asymmetrical braid is soft and has such a gorgeous shape! It's best to start this style with leftover or brushed out 1-inch wand curls.

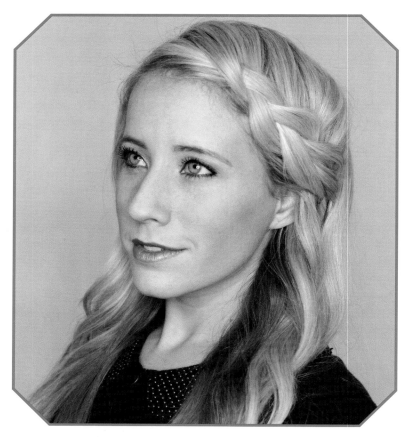

1. Make a deep side part and begin a regular Dutch French Braid. As you're braiding, keep the braid close to your head and angle it toward where you want to tie it off.

2. When you hit your ear, angle the braid back and secure it with a couple of bobby pins. You can use the technique behind the Simple Half-Up (see pages 18–19). and fold the bottom section of the braid over the top and then slide in the bobby pins. After you've secured the braid, go back in and pancake the sections to give your braid so much more definition and texture.

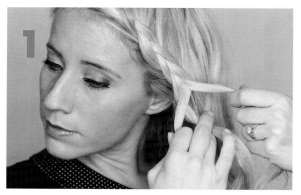

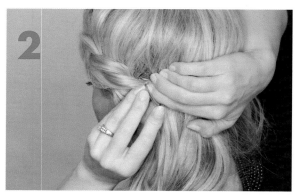

Side Dutch Braid

1. Start with a deep side part.

2. Divide a section of hair near your part into three sections and begin a Dutch French Braid.

3. Continue braiding, making sure to keep the braid tight and close to your hairline.

4. This is what the other side should look like.

5. Bring in those new sections from the opposite side of your head.

6. When you run out of hair to add in, just continue a regular three-strand braid all the way down.

7. Pancake the braid and spread those sections of hair. That is where the style goes from pretty to absolutely stunning. People don't realize it's just you're regular Dutch Braid because the braid is so full and beautiful. After you've pancaked the braid, go ahead and tie it off with a clear elastic band and spray with hair spray.

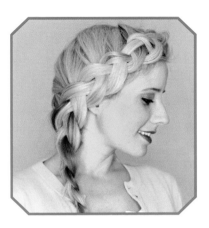

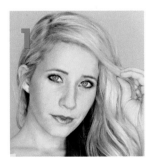
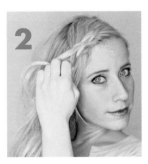
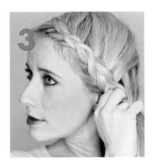
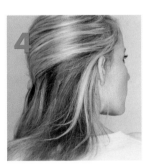

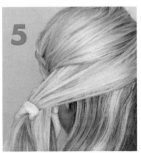
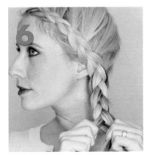
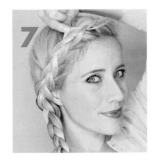

❧ Princess Braids ❧

You are going to create one-sided Dutch Pigtail Braids wrapped in an updo. But instead of adding hair to the top section like you normally would in a Dutch Braid, you are only going to add hair to the bottom section.

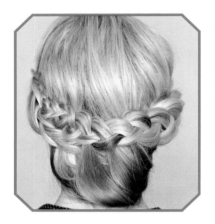

1. Braid a Dutch French Braid down to about the tops of your ears. Pay close attention to what my wrist is doing from step one to step two. In a regular Dutch Braid my next step would be to add a section of hair to that top section.

2. Instead, I'm simply twisting my wrist, which automatically braids that top section underneath the middle section. From here on out you will not be adding hair to the top section of the braid, and it's just easier if you twist your wrist!

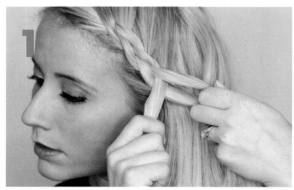

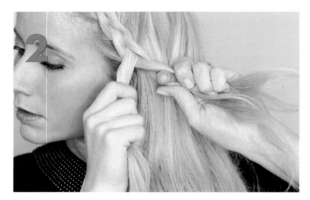

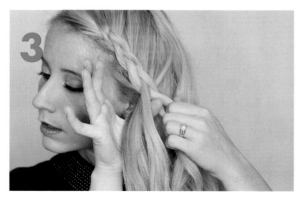

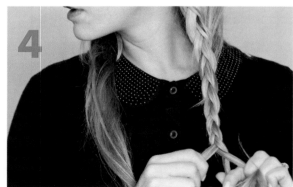

3. Add hair to the bottom section and braid like normal. Braid in the hair that falls forward on your shoulder to that bottom piece. This might take some time getting use to, but with practice you'll be able to get it.

4. When you've run out of hair on one side, continue braiding all the way down and secure with a clear elastic band.

5. Repeat steps 1–4 on the opposite side and then pancake the braids.

6. Take one of the braids and drape it above the nape of your neck. Use large bobby pins to secure the braid to your head. If you have super long hair, you'll need to coil the ends and pin them down so that they can be covered by the next braid.

7. Drape the second braid over the first braid and use large bobby pins to hold in place. The goal is to cover up the ends of the first braid and make sure both braids feel secure.

8. Coil up the ends of the second braid and tuck them behind the first. They should fit nicely in a small pocket. Finish with a firm-hold hair spray. If you need to, take your rattail comb and slide it in horizontally at the crown of your head and lift up to prevent any hair from sticking to your head and give you more volume.

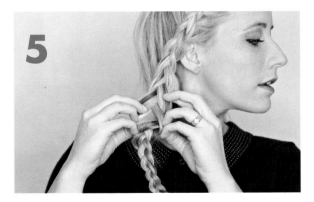

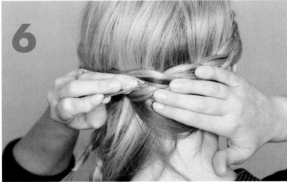

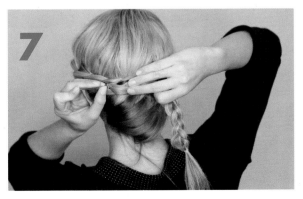

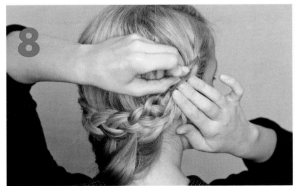

Double-Dutch Pigtail Braids

This is a great style to do on third- or fourth-day hair and when you have loose waves from leftover curls.

1. Split the hair down the center and clip back one of the sides. I like to keep my regular side part on top and just gradually angle it into the center.

2. Take a rather large triangular section from the front. Mine is from about my temples to the end of my part. Separate it into three sections and begin a Dutch French Braid.

3. Dutch French Braid all the way down your head and secure with a couple duckbill clips.

4. Repeat steps 2–3 on the other side.

5. Pancake the braids and spread the sections to add more volume and definition.

6. Combine the braids into a ponytail at the base of your neck and tie them together with an elastic. Remove the clips and unravel the braids below the elastic.

7. Tease the ponytail to add more texture and volume to the hair.

Tip

You can take a small section of hair from underneath the ponytail and wrap it around the elastic. Use a Topsy Tail to secure it inside the ponytail or secure it with a bobby pin underneath the ponytail.

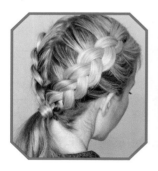
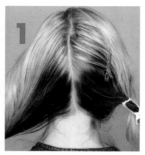
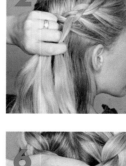
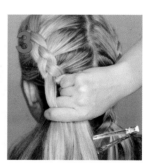
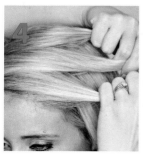
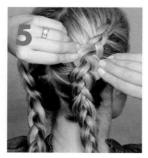
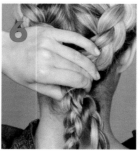
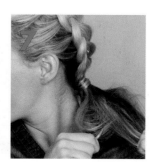

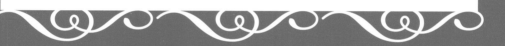

Fishtails

The Fishtail Braid is also known as the Herringbone, the Fish Bone, or the Mermaid Braid. It looks very elaborate but is surprisingly simple. Even though it involves four strands of hair instead of three like in French and Dutch Braids, many people find this style much easier to learn. In general, you want to use the same thickness for each section throughout the braid, and for a more intricate look use skinnier strands. It takes more effort and time, but it will look absolutely gorgeous.

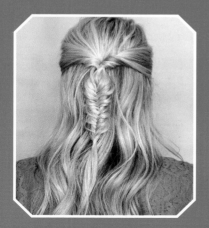
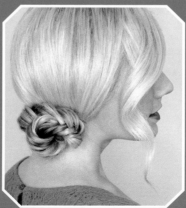
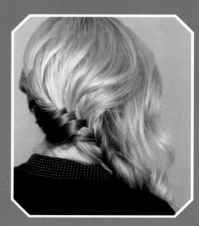

~Side Fishtail~

The Fishtail Braid is classic. These steps show it on the side, but they apply for any position. I love styling it with messy, textured hair as it gives the braid a nice full look. This is a style that works well on third- or fourth-day hair!

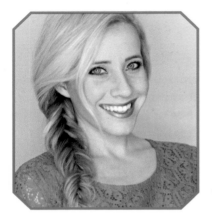

1. Gather your hair in a low side ponytail and tie it off using a clear elastic. Split the tail into two sections.

2. Using your index finger, split off a small section of hair from the right section.

3. Point your index finger toward the left section.

4. Grab that small section and incorporate it into the left section.

5. Using your index finger, split off a small section of hair from the left section.

6. Point your index finger toward the right section.

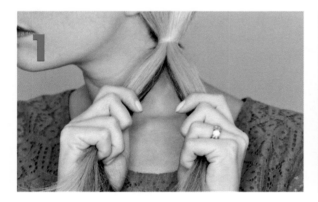

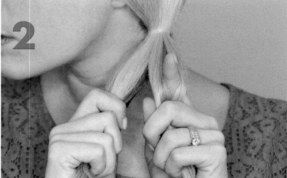

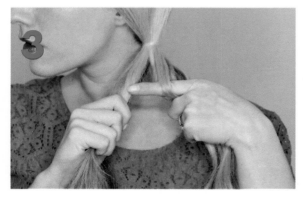

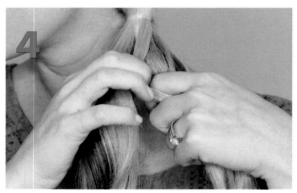

7. Incorporate that small section into the right section. You will start seeing your fishtail form. Make sure to keep the strands tight as you can always go in and loosen them later.

8. Continue braiding down the hair.

9. Tie off the fishtail braid and cut out the elastic up top, making sure to not snip your hair.

10. Now you're going to pancake your fishtail. You can leave it nice and tight or pull out some of the layers to make it look a little more effortless. It's all personal preference.

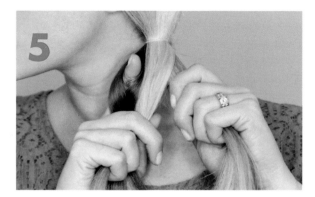

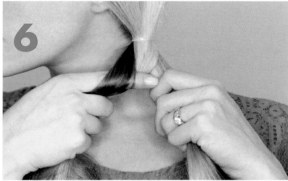

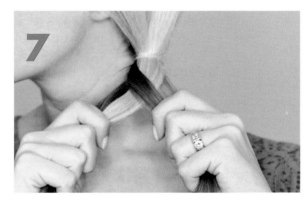

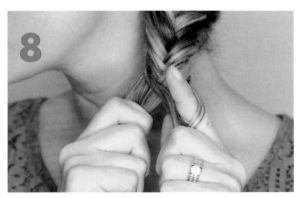

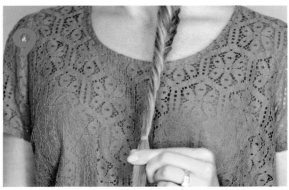

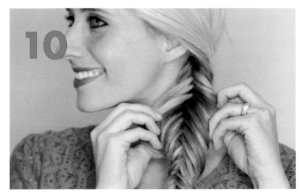

French Fishtail

You must be familiar with a regular Fishtail Braid to make any sense out of this tutorial. Once you get that, it'll be easy peasy!

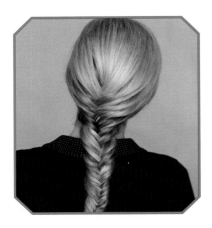

1. Gather a small section of hair. Where you decide to gather this section is where your Fishtail Braid will start.

2. Split the hair into two sections.

3. Holding both sections in your left hand, section off a small piece of hair from the back of the right section with your right hand.

4. Using your left hand, reach over the right section and grab that small piece of hair. Pull it over the right section and combine it with the left section.

5. Move both sections into your right hand and section off a small piece of hair from the back of the left section with your left hand.

6. Using your right hand, reach over the left section and grab that small piece of hair. Pull it over the left section and combine it with the right.

7. Now you're going to start incorporating new hair. Note: You will be moving from the back to the front with these new sections. The sections will be about half an inch thick depending on how textured you want your braid, and you're going to sweep them down and over. So with your right hand section off a small piece of new hair.

8. Sweep that section over the right section and add it to the left. Make sure you are pulling the strands tight. You can always go in and loosen things up afterward.

9. Transfer both sections into your right hand and gather a new section with your left hand.

10. Sweep the new small section over the left section and combine it with the right.

11. Repeat steps 7–9.

12. Right around here is where my arms start turning into jelly, so I move the braid forward onto my shoulder and start Fishtailing the opposite way.

13. Tie off the braid with a clear elastic. Pancake the braid by gently spreading the sections. Doing this will make your braid look thicker and it will add volume and texture.

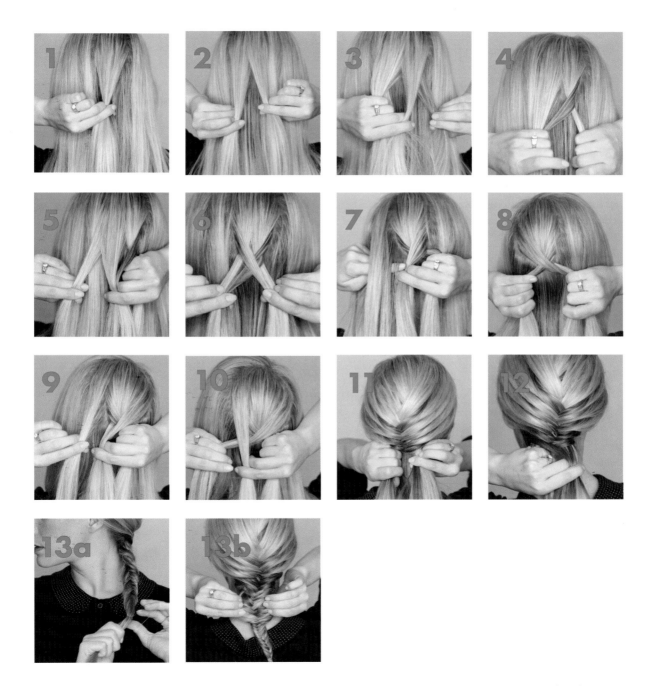

Red-Carpet Style

Start this style off with some pretty curls. You can use the 1-inch wand tutorial on pages 22–23. If you have extensions, this would be a great style to use them on.

1. Part of the charm behind this style is having the perfect Ariel bangs. To get them, wrap your bangs around two fingers toward your face and secure with duckbill clips. You really want to set those curls so that they don't fall out toward the end of the night.

2. Pull your hair half up. I've used the Simple Half-Up technique on pages 18–19 where you fold the hair and then slide the bobby pin up through the seam. I secured the hair off center.

3. Take a chunk of hair from the nape of your neck and clip the rest of the hair out of the way using a large butterfly clip. Divide that chunk into two sections and Fishtail it all the way down.

4. When you've finished your Fishtail, pancake it to make it look messy and random. You want a very effortless look here.

5. Instead of tying off with a clear elastic band, tease the ends of the Fishtail and spray with hair spray. This will hold the Fishtail in place all night.

6. Release the rest of the hair from the butterfly clip and add in more volume to the curls by teasing with a rattail comb.

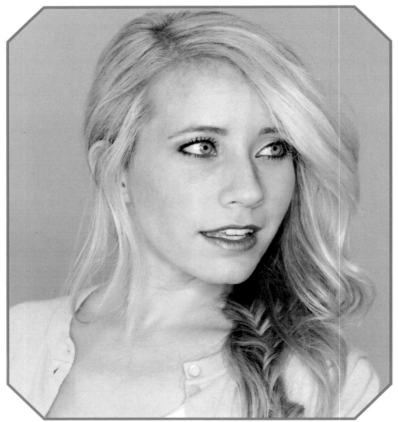

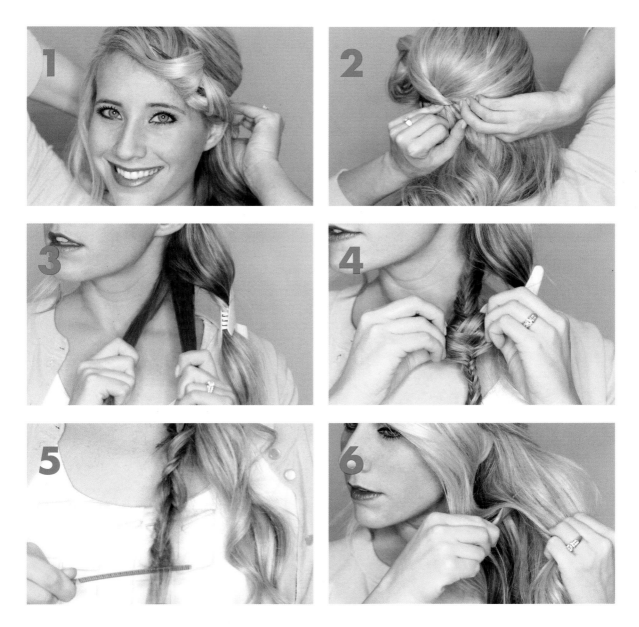

Elegance Swept to the Side

You will need to be familiar with the French Fishtail and the Alternative Braid. Please refer to those tutorials on pages 60–61 and 31 for more in-depth instructions. You want fresh falling curls for this style made from the 1-inch wand tutorial, which can be found on pages 22–23. Make sure to tease your hair to add volume and set the hairstyle with firm hold hair spray to finish it off.

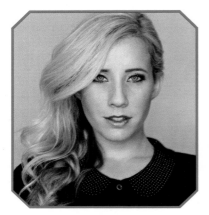

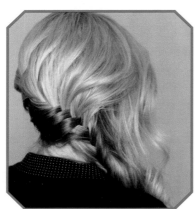

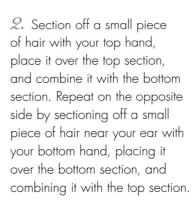

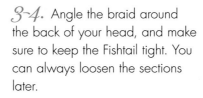

1. Gather the section of hair from your ear to the end of your part and secure it with a clear elastic band. Divide the tail into two sections. These two sections will start the French Fishtail Braid. Make sure you don't incorporate those front sections of hair into your braid, as you want the fresh curls in front to help finish off the look (see step 7).

2. Section off a small piece of hair with your top hand, place it over the top section, and combine it with the bottom section. Repeat on the opposite side by sectioning off a small piece of hair near your ear with your bottom hand, placing it over the bottom section, and combining it with the top section.

3-4. Angle the braid around the back of your head, and make sure to keep the Fishtail tight. You can always loosen the sections later.

5. When you get to the nape of your neck you're going to section off the front curls (refer to step 7). and begin an Alternative Braid.

6. Split the hair into two sections and twirl them inward.

7. Combine the twists and push your finger through the sections to produce two new sections. Twirl the sections inward, and repeat step 7.

8. Tie off the Alternative Braid using a clear elastic band.

9. Pancake the braid by tugging on some of the sections to add extra volume and texture to the braid. Cut out the elastic band holding the Fishtail together, and either leave the elastic holding the Alternative Braid in or take it out and tease the ends really well. If you do this and spray them with hair spray, the braid will stay put all night.

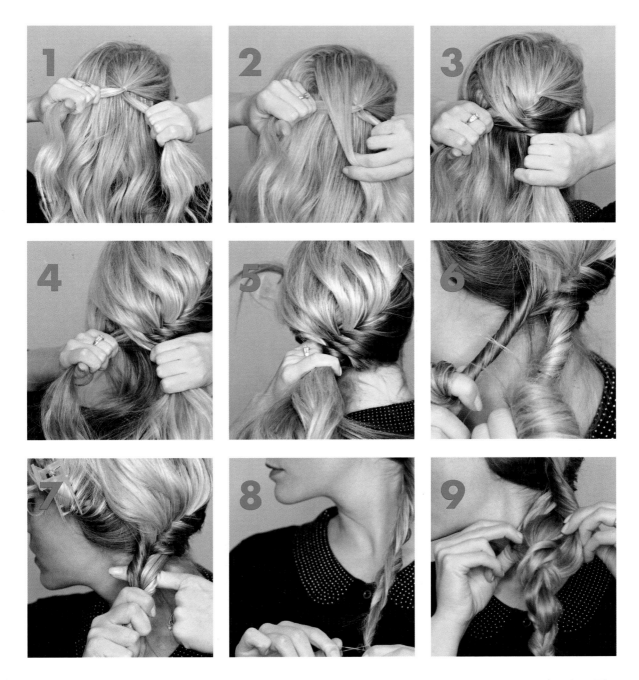

Half-Up Fishtail

I started this style by curling my hair with a 1-inch curling wand. Tutorial on pages 22–23.

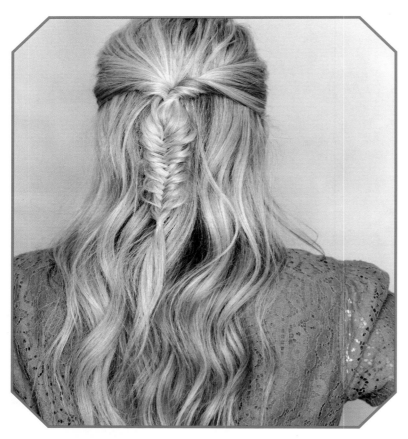

1–2. Pull half the hair up into an elastic band. You don't want to pull all the thickness up, just those very top layers. You can either use a Topsy Tail for this next part or create a hole above the elastic and pull your tail up, over, and through the hole.

3–7. Divide the tail into two sections and begin your Fishtail Braid. You should be familiar with this braid by now but if you need a refresher, head on over to pages 58–59 and we'll get you taken care of!

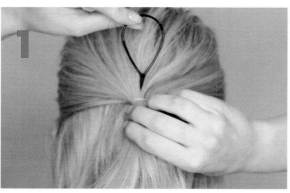

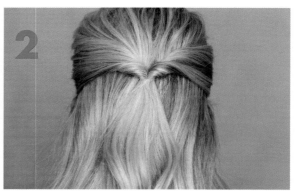

8. When you are finished, tie off the Fishtail with a clear elastic band and then pancake the braid. This is where you get to bring in your own creativity. You can either make it look super bohemian and random, or you can leave it looking straighter and more refined.

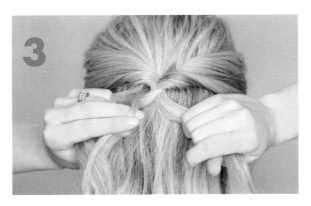

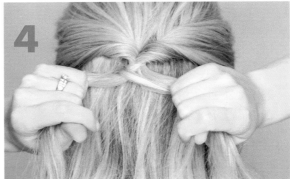

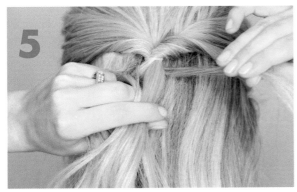

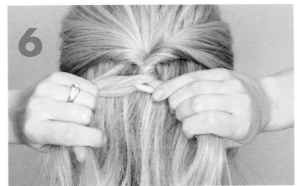

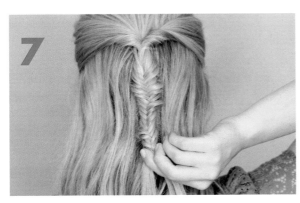

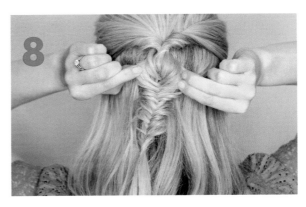

~Fishtail Bun~

1. Split the hair into two sections. Tie each off with a clear elastic band one inch away from your part.

2. Fishtail one of the tails.

3. Pancake it to make it look fuller.

4. Repeat on the other side, and then hide the part by loosening some of the hair above each ponytail.

5. There are a couple different ways you can finish off this Fishtail Bun. The first way is to wrap the tails in a circular direction. One Fishtail goes over and around the other one, and then the other one starts and you're just basically pinning the tails into a circle.

OR

6. The other way is create a figure eight with the Fishtails. Instead of going all the way over and around the other Fishtail, you'll bring it around and through the center space.

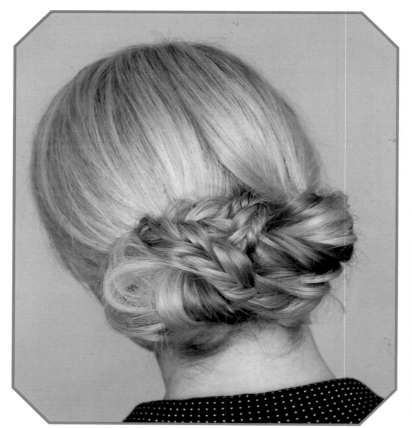

Tip

Keep playing with the tails until you get the shape you want. Make sure to use enough bobby pins that the style holds. I prefer using large bobby pins as opposed to regular sized ones.

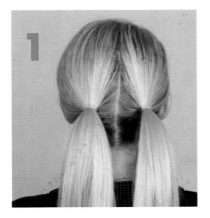
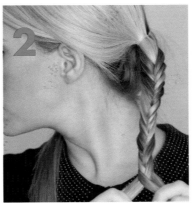
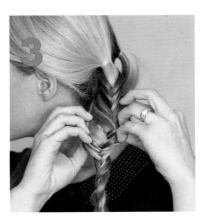
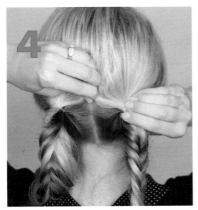
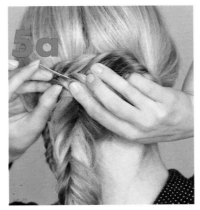
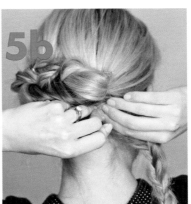
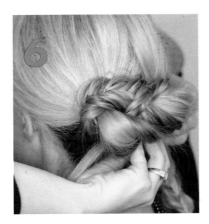

Fishtail Side Bun

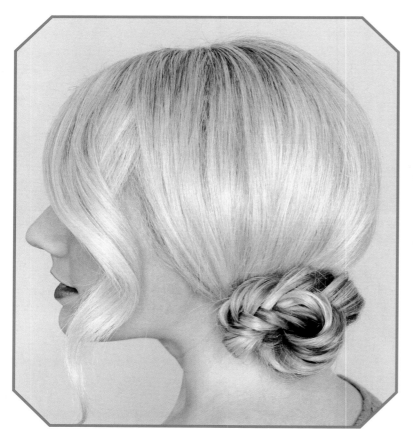

1. Complete steps 1–8 of the Side Fishtail on pages 58–59. Start by pulling the hair into a side ponytail and Fishtail all the way down. Tie it off with a clear elastic band and then pancake the braid to make it look fuller.

2. Simply wrap your Fishtail toward your face and create an upside down C shape with your braid. Secure with bobby pins as you go, and finish with firm-hold hair spray.

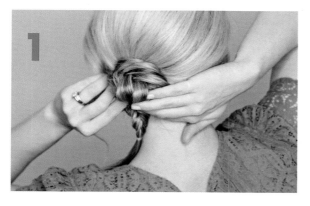

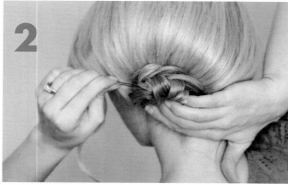

Ponytails

A ponytail is certainly the easiest and fastest way to get your hair up and out of your face. It comes in handy when you're rushed in the mornings, you need your hair off your neck to exercise, or you want to show off that gorgeous face of yours. Because a plain old ponytail doesn't require much effort, it tends to be overused and abused. Hopefully these next hairstyles will spark some creativity and help you upcycle the humble tail.

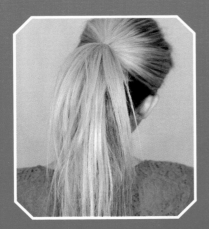
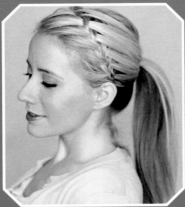
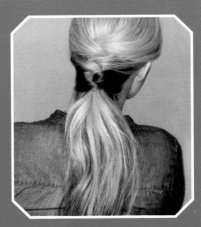

Crisscross Ponytail

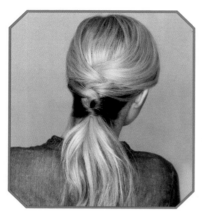

1. Gather a small section of hair from the front.

2. Combine it with a thin section of hair from the back and tie off with a clear elastic band.

3. Take a small section from the opposite side and combine it with another thin section of hair from the back.

4. Using a clear elastic, combine the sections.

5. Repeat until you have four crisscrosses. Leave out two small sections near the nape of your neck, and tie the rest of your hair into a ponytail.

6. Wrap the right section over the ponytail and then wrap the left section over the ponytail. You'll need to hold these sections tight with your free hand.

7. Secure the sections with a clear elastic band underneath the ponytail. You can try sliding them into the existing elastic band or just use a new one.

Tip

You don't need to tie the elastic bands super tightly. You just want the elastics to loosely hold the hair in place. When you remove the elastics, gently slide them out of your hair.

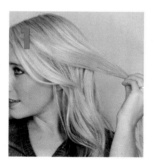
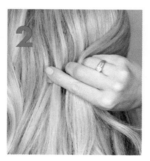
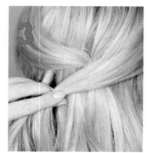
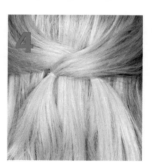

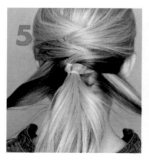
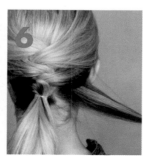
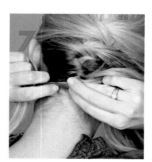

Formal Ponytail

1. Place your index fingers right above your ears and gently pull back the top layers of hair. When the sections meet, begin folding them. (See Simple Half-Up on pages 18–19).

2–3. Fold the hair over itself and slide a bobby pin into the fold to secure the hair, pinning only the outer layers of hair.

4. Gently pull back two more sections of hair from the front. These sections are going to be much thinner than the first two, and it's important to recognize that I'm only folding those small sections, not the entire layer of hair.

5. With the flat side of your bobby pin on top, push the bobby pin into the fold. The goal of this hairstyle is to have a really gorgeous seam of folded hair. You can make it a vertical seam or an angled seam. I like to angle mine as it's easier to hide any mistakes and I just really love the look of it. So keep that in mind as you're pinning the sections below.

6. Continue taking small sections, folding them back, and pinning them in place. When you reach the nape of your neck, take one last section from only one side and hold in place with your finger.

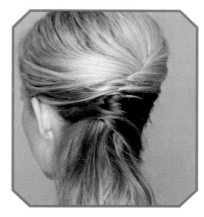

7. Replace your finger with a bobby pin and tease the ponytail to make it look even more voluminous.

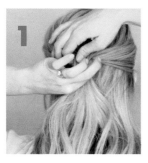
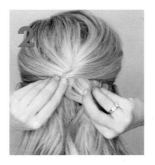
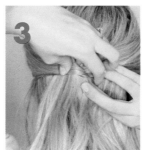
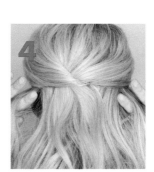
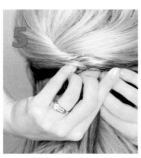
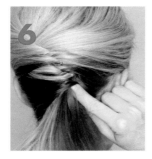
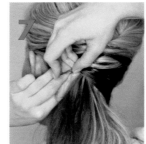

Waterfall Ponytail

This is such a fun and unique hairstyle! I love that the Waterfall Braid creates a beautiful headband. If you understand how to Waterfall Braid, it will only take you a second or two to figure out how to braid it at a different angle. You can dress this style up and make it look super fancy, or it can be very casual.

1. Make a deep side part and section off the front headband area. Pull the rest of the hair back to get it out of the way.

2. Begin a Waterfall Braid (see pages 42–43) by dividing a small layer of hair into three sections.

3. Braid once: front piece over middle, back piece over middle. Drop that very back piece.

4. Use a duckbill clip to clip that back piece out of the way. Replace that back piece with another section of hair and continue braiding.

5. Braid that new section over the middle and then add a new section of hair to the front piece.

6. Braid that over the middle, transfer the sections into your front hand, and drop that back piece.

7. Add that dropped section into your duckbill clip and continue on with your waterfall braid.

8. When you get to the opposite ear, push a bobby pin into the braid to secure it down.

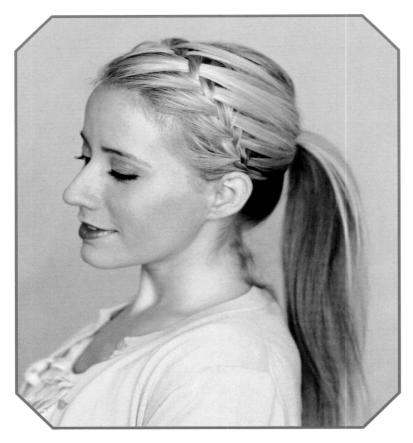

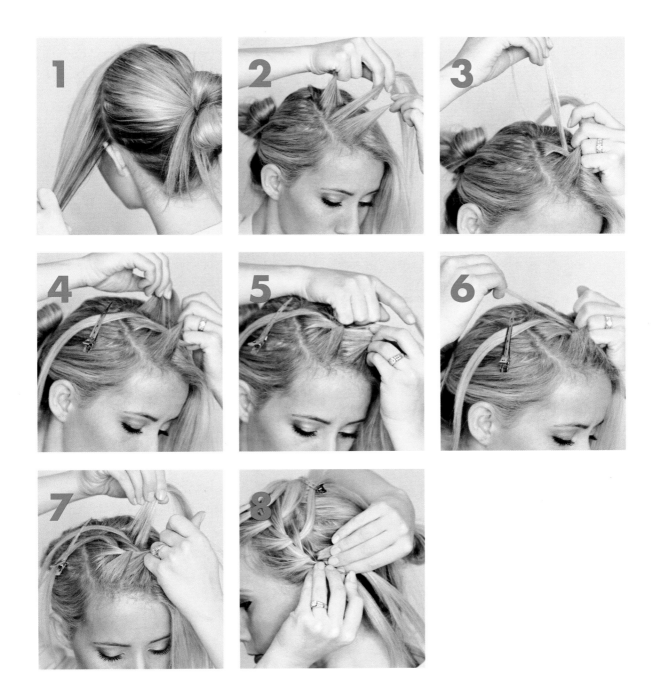

The Perfect Ponytail

This is a great trick for making your average ponytail look super-glam!
Not only does it add length, but it also creates height and volume.

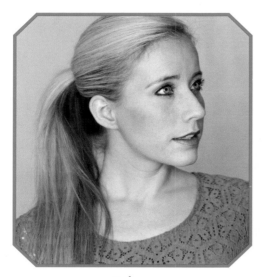

Before

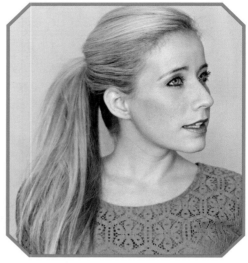

After

1. Section off the top half of hair by securing it with a large butterfly clip. Tie the bottom section into a ponytail with a clear elastic band.

2. Smooth out the top section and gather it into a ponytail about an inch or two above the first ponytail. Secure it with a clear elastic band.

3. Tease and spray the top ponytail with a firm-hold hair spray. Once you've brushed out the snarls, tighten the ponytail. Viola!

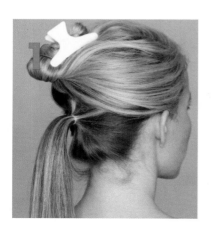

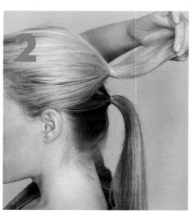

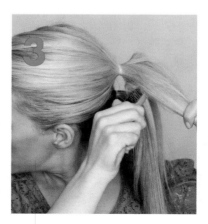

Formal

Have a special event coming up? I've got you covered. Whether it's for a prom, a wedding, or even a red carpet, you'll be feeling glamorous in no time. In this section you'll find fabulous tricks and tips to achieve some truly beautiful and elegant hairstyles. From a classic French Twist to Bohemian Updos, I'll take you through all the steps you need to achieve the perfect style to make you feel gorgeous and chic for whatever magical night awaits you.

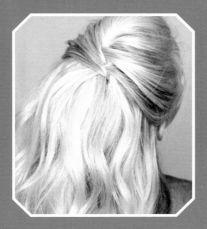
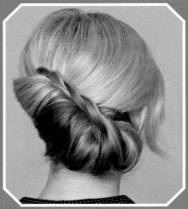
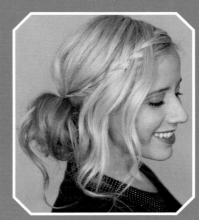

Twisted Chignon

This is one of my favorite hairstyles. It's so neat and polished looking, but it has such a gorgeous shape, so it's still fun and feminine. I also love that you don't need any curls to make this hairstyle work. Granted, every hairstyle looks better with some curls in it, but if you're in a hurry to look nice and you don't have extra time to spend on curling your hair, this is the perfect style!

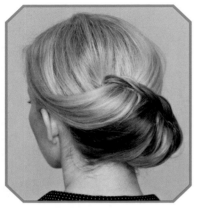

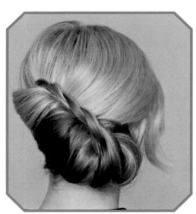

1. Take a section of hair from one side of the front and pin it in the back by sliding your bobby pin in horizontally. Slide in another bobby pin, crisscrossing the two.

2. Take another small section of hair from the same side of the front and repeat.

3. Take a section of hair from behind your ear on the opposite side and begin rolling it around two fingers. Pin that roll to your head by sliding in a bobby pin where your finger starts, angling it up and toward the side the hair came from.

4. Continue taking small sections of hair and guiding them with your fingers and thumb into a nicely shaped roll. Pin as you go, and make sure to cover that first set of bobby pins we put up in steps 1 and 2.

5. If there is an obvious hole or gap at the bottom of your twist, take a small section near the nape of your neck and twist it up to hide the gap. Secure with bobby pins. Large bobby pins may come in handy!

6. Take the rest of the hair that's still down, and divide it into two equal sections.

7. Loosely twist the sections of hair together, and fluff them up using a rattail comb. Secure with a clear elastic band.

8. Take that twist up and over the pinned hair, placing it gently on top of the seam. When you get to the other side, tuck the ends down inside the hole of the first roll. Using this twist to finish off the style not only adds interest but also hides any gaps or pins from the previous steps.

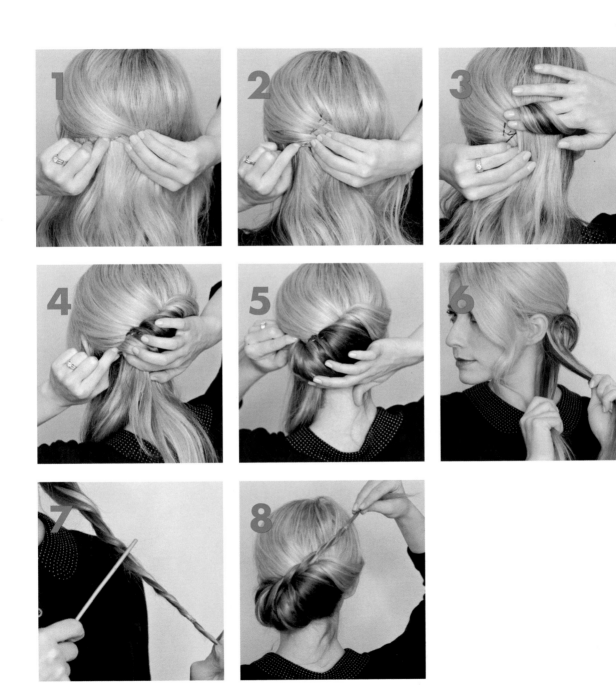

Twisted Updo

1. Section out your bangs and then tie off the hair from your ears up to where the back of your part ends. Pull the rest into a low Fast Messy Bun (see pages 92–93). The shape of this Fast Messy Bun is very important as it gives shape to the rest of the hairstyle. If you're not in love with your bun, try it again until you are.

2. Take out two sections from the hair you tied up. You will only be using one at a time, but I wanted to show you what the front looks like before moving to the back.

3. Gently twist and pancake one section of hair. You can twist the entire section away from your face, or you can split it into two sections and twist them around each other. Either way works.

4. Drape that twisted section over the Messy Bun and secure on the opposite side with bobby pins. If your hair is long, you'll need to coil up the ends and secure with another bobby pin like in step 6.

5. Gently twist and drape the other section over the bun and secure with bobby pins.

6. Repeat these steps until you run out of hair from that top section you tied off. Make sure to alternate sides, drape loosely, and hide any visible pins with the next section of hair.

7. Push the ends of that last section inside the gap between the draped section and your head. Finish off with firm-hold hair spray and pull out fringe around your temples and ears and any bangs you wish to have out.

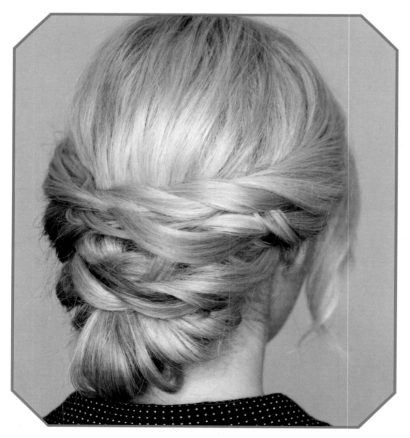

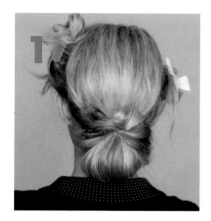 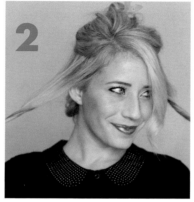 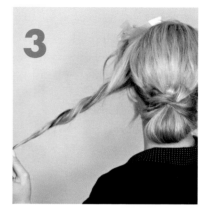

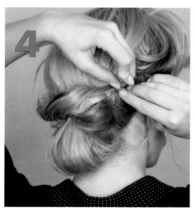 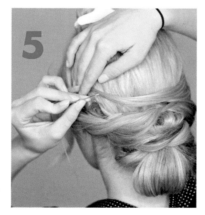 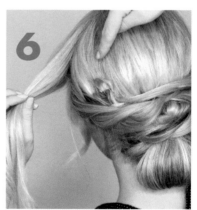

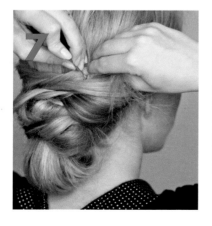

Tip

You don't need to have curly hair for this hairstyle to work, although you'll get a prettier shape if you have some sort of texture in your hair. I started with four-day-old, 1-inch wand curls.

Waterfall Updo

Start this style with 1-inch wand curls and teased roots. If you need to brush up on your Waterfall Braid technique, see pages 42–43.

1. Section off the front layers of hair on the heaviest side of your part. I've sectioned off only a few inches back from my forehead.

2. Tie the remaining hair into an upside down bun, meaning that on your last pass through just simply flip the ends up.

3. Create whatever shape you'd like with the bun.

4. I wanted something very elegant looking and I think it's very pretty when you have the Waterfall'ed section from the front meeting with hair that's Waterfall'ing out of the bun. Get creative and be patient getting that perfect bun.

5. Gather a layer of hair near the part and start a Waterfall Braid. Divide the hair into three sections, pull the back section over the middle, then pull the front section over the middle section, move all three strands into your front hand, and add a new section of hair to the back section. Braid the back section over the middle, transfer all three strands to the back hand, then drop that bottom piece. Replace the section you dropped with a new one, and braid it over the middle.

6. Continue these steps until you reach the end.

7. Wrap the Waterfall Braid around the bun and secure with a bobby pin.

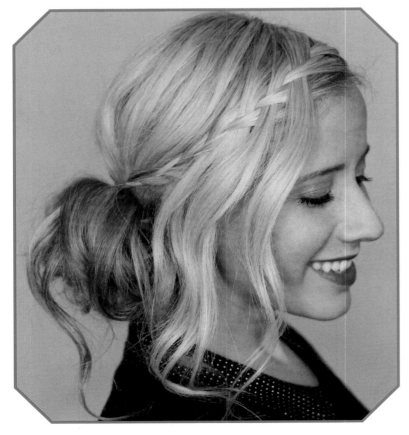

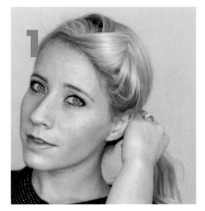 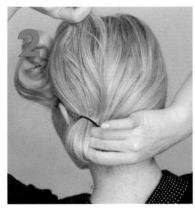 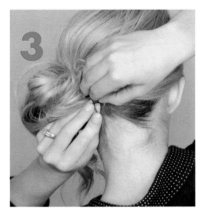

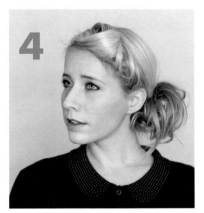 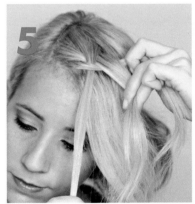 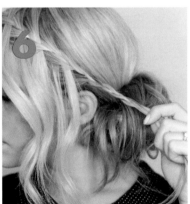

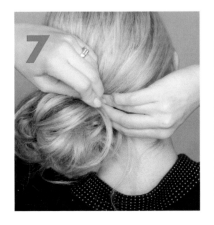

Tips

Finish this style off by spraying with a firm-hold hair spray. If you feel it's a little snug to your head, insert the end of a rattail comb into your hair and pull up. This will loosen the hair around your head and give you a little bit more volume.

Twisted Bohemian Updo

This style works best on dirty, textured hair because the pins can grip a little bit better and the hair is easier to manipulate. I used leftover 1-inch wand curls and found that having those big bouncy curls made creating the shape of the bun much easier.

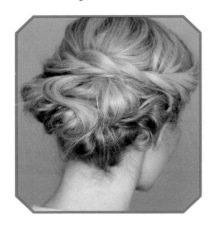 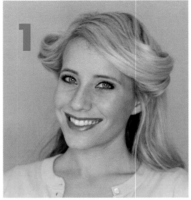 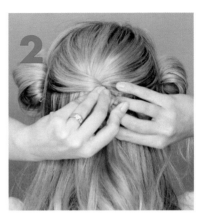

1. Roll, clip, or tie the front sections of hair out of the way as you'll be using them later on.

2. Gently pull your hair half up. If you need a quick refresher, the Simple Half-Up tutorial is on pages 18–19.

3. Tease the bottom layers of hair.

4. This next part is completely random with the goal of creating a pretty shape by taking chunks of hair and pinning them to the head.

5. Continue pinning up all the hair off the neck, making sure it doesn't look too messy but has a great shape.

6. Now that all your hair is off your neck, release those front sections. Take a small section near your part and divide it into two sections.

7. Begin twisting the hair away from the face.

8. You'll add in more layers of hair as you twist down, but there's no technique behind this. Just twist and add in more hair where needed. Be sure to angle your twist back, or else you might end up with some funky bubbles.

9. Once you've reached the end of the twist, tie them off with a clear elastic band and then fluff up the twist with a rattail comb. This will give the twist some texture and definition.

10. Next drape the twist across the back of your head and directly on top of the bun.

11. Repeat steps 6–10 on the opposite side.

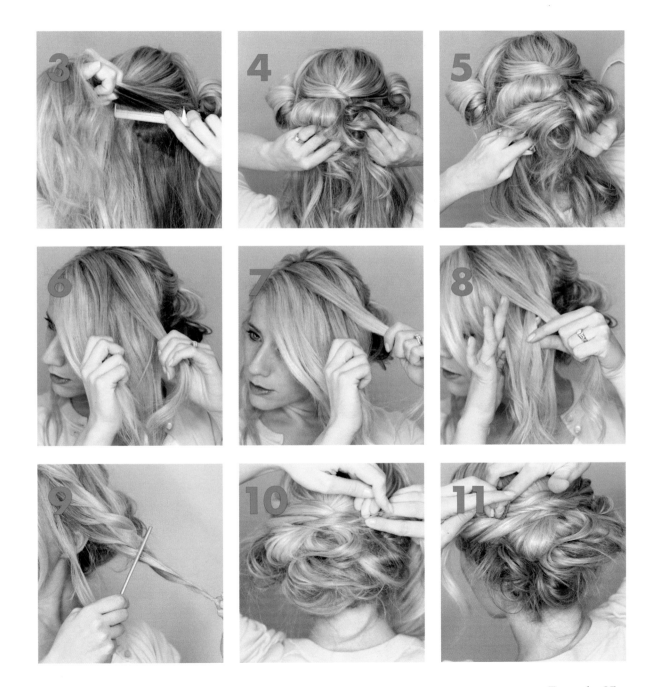

Simple Headband Updo

This is such a fun, easy style that you can dress up or down depending on the headband you use!

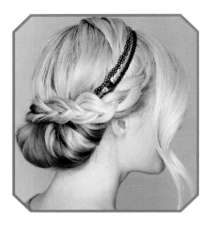

1. Place a headband around the crown of your head. It's important that the band isn't too loose or too tight.

2. Pull forward hair from an inch behind each ear. Clip the hair in front.

3. Secure the hair in back, a few inches from the ends, using a clear elastic band.

4. Hold onto the elastic with your dominant hand and roll the hair into the headband.

5. Tuck the ends into the headband. Spray with hair spray. Take a thin section from the front and gently twist it back. Lay the twist on top of the rolled hair and secure on the other side with bobby pins.

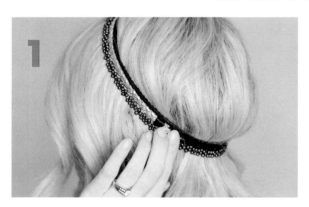

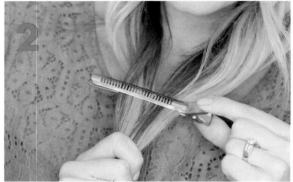

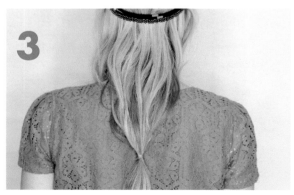

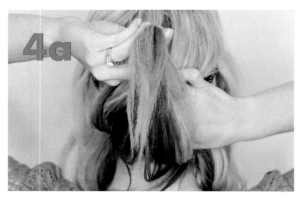

6. On the other side and behind the bangs (if you want to leave them out), divide the hair into three sections and Dutch French Braid. Remember, the outer sections go OVER the middle.

7. Keep the braid tight and angle it back, this way when you drape it over the twist it will lay nicely. Pancake and tie off the braid with a clear elastic band.

8. Gently drape the braid over the twist.

9. Secure the ends by tucking them into the headband.

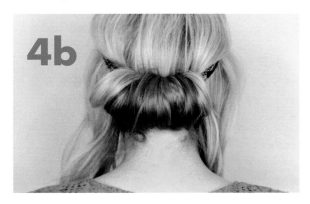

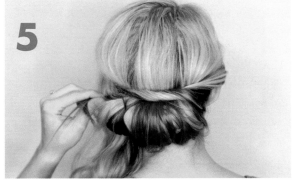

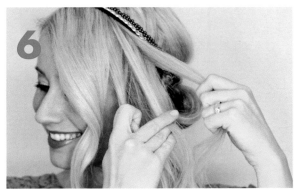

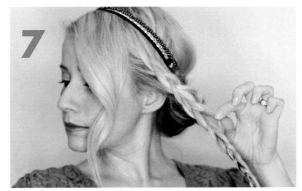

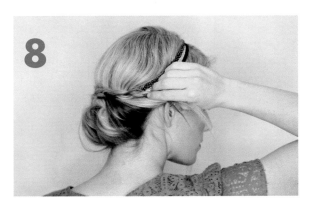

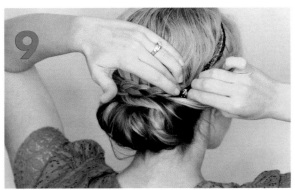

Crisscross Half-Up

This is a great hairstyle for second- or third- day hair because the more grip and texture you have in your hair, the stronger the pins are going to hold. I've started this style with 1-inch curls (see page 22–23).

1. Rough up your part with your fingers, then tease back your bangs to give you more volume and height.

2. Pin back that front section into a Pompadour and spray it with firm spray hair spray. For more instructions see page 20.

3. Gather two thin sections of hair from the sides directly below your Pompadour.

4. Fold the sections over themselves and insert a bobby pin into the seam. Make sure to cover up any pins from the Pompadour.

5. Gather two more thin sections of hair. Fold the sections over themselves and pin the seam. In order for the crisscrosses to show, pin each fold a little behind and off center from the one before it.

6. Take the remaining hair that's down and tease it to create that big, bouncy shape.

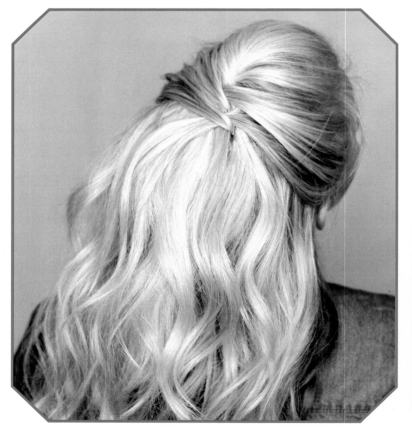

Tip

You're not pinning huge sections of hair, just the layers in the very front and on top, so one or two bobby pins should easily hold the hair in place.

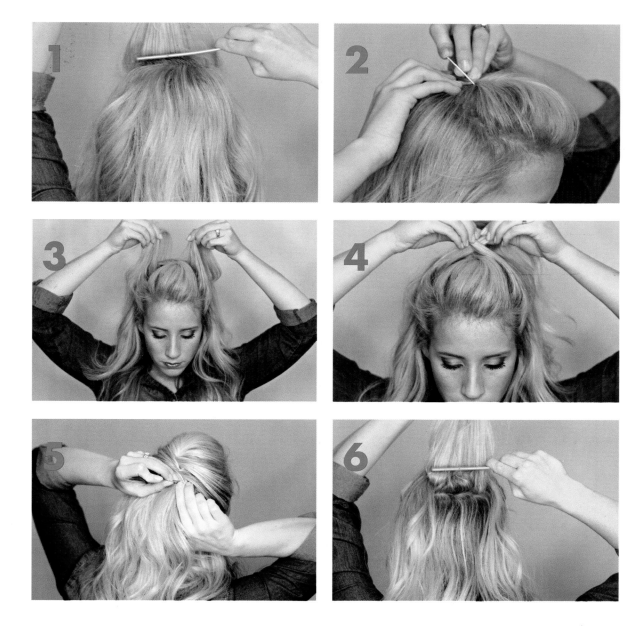

Crisscross French Twist

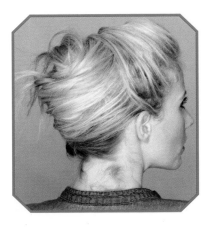

1. Follow the instructions on page 88–89 to create a Crisscross Half-Up.

2. Pull your hair back as if you were going to tie it up in a ponytail.

3. Begin twisting the base of the ponytail toward your face.

4. Hold the twist tight, then angle it vertically.

5. Start pinning the twist to your head by inserting bobby pins into the fold. Pin a tiny bit of hair from the twist, then push the pin in deeper so it can grab the hair underneath the twist. Continue twisting and pinning until you get to the top of your head.

6. Pin down some ends that are sticking out. Get creative! I love the look of the classic French Twist with modern messy ends.

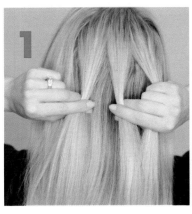

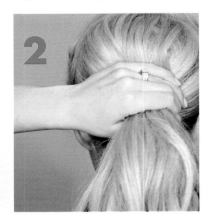

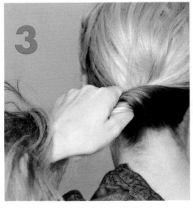

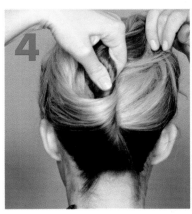

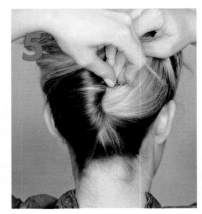

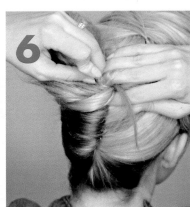

Buns

Buns are all the rage right now! They're so versatile, and they can be easily dressed up for a night out, or down for a trip to the store. In this next chapter I'll be sharing some of my favorite ways to style a bun, whether it be braided, banded, or bohemian. Hopefully you'll be inspired along the way to start thinking a little further outside the box when it comes to styling your hair! Remember, you can share your gorgeous 'dos on Instagram, tagged @twistmepretty.

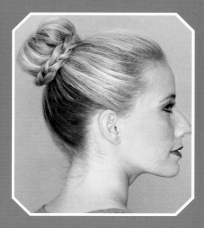 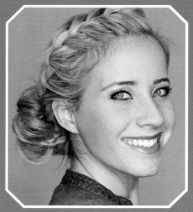 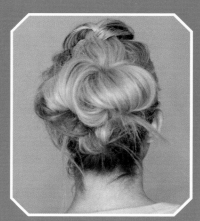

Fast Messy Bun

The thing about random hairstyles like this is that sometimes they work on the first try and you love the shape, and other times they just don't! So if you're not getting that perfect shape, just pull it out and start over.

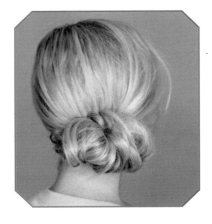

1. Tease the roots and brush out any visible snarls. Gather your hair into a low side ponytail, and wrap an elastic band once around your gathered hair.

2. Twist the band.

3. Begin pulling the hair through the band as if you were going to tie a ponytail.

4. Instead of pulling the ponytail all the way through the elastic, you're going to sweep your fingers underneath the hair.

5. Reach up and find the bulk of the bun and grab it with that same hand.

6-7. Once your hand is on the bulk of the bun, take your other hand and finish the rotation of the band buy pulling it off your hand and over your hair.

8. You should be left with a random little bun.

9. Two bobby pins transformed the previous step into this bun. I simply grabbed a small section of that larger bun area, pulled it up, and pinned it to my head. Play around with the bun until you get the shape you want and pin it in place.

Tip

Fast Messy Buns are fabulous! If you're having a terrible hair day and your curls are crazy, or you slept like a wild animal the night before and have just a mess of strands going on, the Fast Messy Bun is the perfect hairstyle for you. It hides stray pieces and makes your messy hair look very intentional. I love the shape of Fast Messy Buns, and my favorite way to wear them is low and to the side.

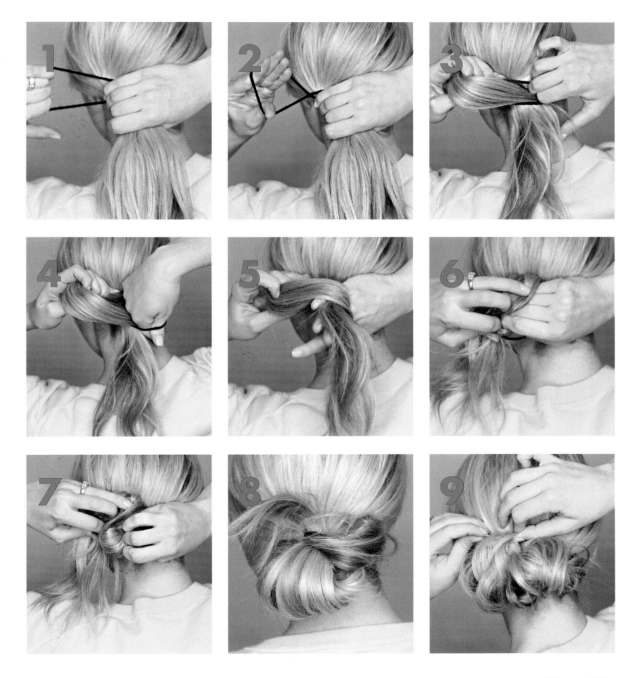

Three-Banded Bun

This style is so easy even though it looks super intricate. I promise if you wear your hair like this, everyone will be complimenting you and asking you how in the world you did it. It's such a fun style for early mornings and dirty hair! In order to create this look you need to be familiar with how to create a good Fast Messy Bun (see pages 92–93) as this style is simply three Fast Messy Buns that end up looking like one!

1. You will be dividing the hair into three equal sections. Your first step is to gather a section and then drape the rest of your hair over your shoulder to get it out of the way.

2. Tie gathered section into a Fast Messy Bun.

3. Gather the middle of section hair and tie it into a Fast Messy Bun.

4. Gather the last section of hair and tie it into a Fast Messy Bun.

5. To make sure the three messy buns look like one large section, hide any holes by pinning the sections of hair together with bobby pins and create that perfect shape!

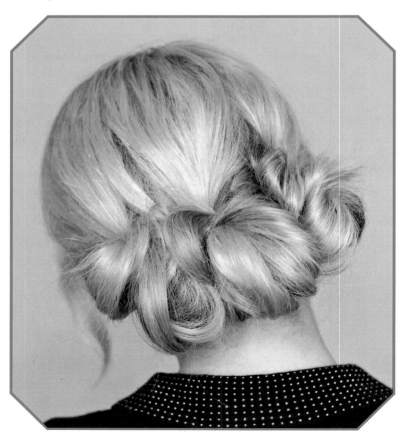

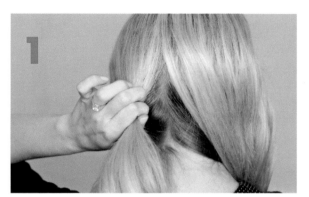

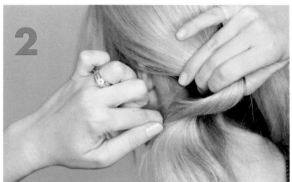

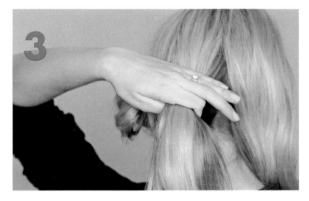

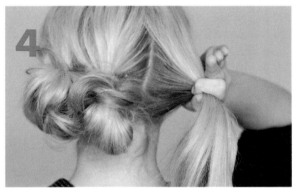

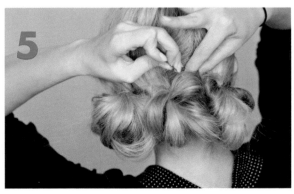

French Braided Messy Bun

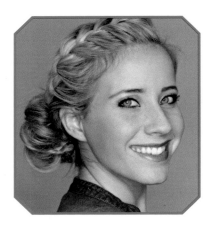

1. Start with a side part and begin French Braiding down to your ear. Remember, in a regular French Braid the two outermost sections go over the middle section.

2. When you reach your ear, finish off the section with a three-strand braid and secure it with a clear elastic band.

3. I like to pancake just those back sections. By pulling up on the strands it'll give you more volume and height and also making your braid look gorge!

4. Throw your tail into a Fast Messy Bun. A tutorial for that is on pages 92–93.

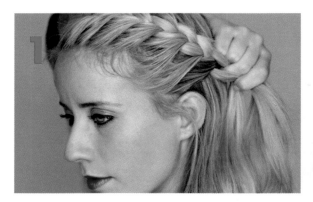

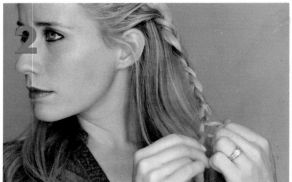

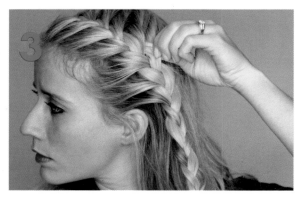

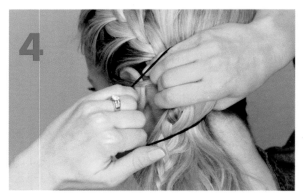

French Braided Pompadour

1. Gather a section of hair from the front and French Braid back. I like to use the outside corners of my eyebrows as a guide.

2. Secure the braid by inserting two horizontal crisscrossing bobby pins.

3. Pull the rest of the hair up into a ponytail.

4. Take a rattail comb and fluff up the ponytail.

5-6. Take your hand and push the ends of your ponytail up inside the elastic band. This is completely messy and random. You can leave some of the ends of your ponytail hanging out like I did, or you can tie it up nice and tight!

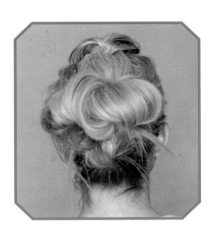

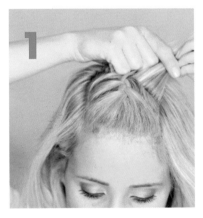

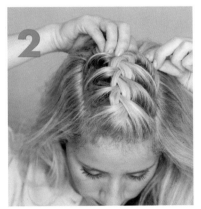

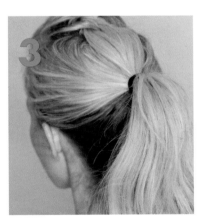

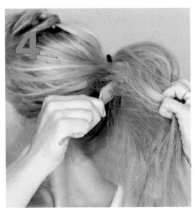

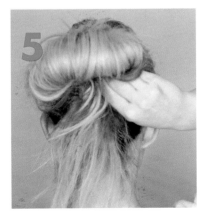

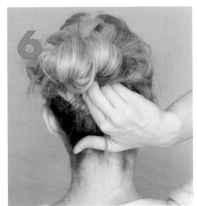

Braided Ballerina Bun

You're going to need a bun former and know how to do a one-sided Dutch French Braid. If you don't have a bun former, chop the toes off a tube sock and roll it up and you'll be good to go! Let's get to it, shall we?

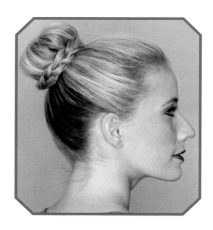

1. This is a bun former; it looks like a donut! I'm using a dark color so you can clearly see it. When you're at the store, though, find one that matches your hair color.

2. Gather your hair up in a high pony, and put your ponytail through the hole of the bun former. It should rest at the base of your ponytail.

3. Drape your hair over the bun former.

4. Tie a thin elastic over the bun former. This will get all the hair out of the way and give you a clear path to braid.

5. Take a small section of hair from the front and divide it into three sections.

6. Now you're going to braid the strand that's closest to your head (the bottom strand) under the middle, and the section that closest to your bun (the top strand) under the middle.

7. Add a new section of hair to the bottom strand, braid it under the middle section, and braid the top section under the middle WITHOUT adding any new hair.

8. Continue braiding the hair around the bun. Right about here is where you'll need to bring your arms forward and begin braiding up.

9. Once you have no hair left to add in, continue a three strand braid until you run out of hair. Tie off with a clear elastic.

10. Put your non-dominant hand over the bun and with your dominant hand remove the thin elastic. You are basically transferring the elastic from your bun to your wrist.

11. Optional: if you want a thicker braid, go ahead and pancake it by spreading apart and pulling on the sections.

12. Now we're going to secure the braid by wrapping it around the bun, as far as it will go, and then tuck the ends of the braid up inside the elastic that's holding your ponytail. Finish this style off by spraying down any flyaways. If you have a bunch of those annoying little hairs at the nape of your neck, comb them into the hair and pin them down. You can pull out any fringe, and if you have straight across bangs please leave them down! Oh so pretty!

Quick refresher course: For a Dutch French Braid you braid the outer sections under the middle section instead of over like in a regular French Braid. As for making it one sided . . . well, that just means you only add a new section of hair to one side instead of both.

Keep the braid as tight and as close to the base of the bun as possible. There's nothing like going through all the steps only to end up with a braid that's too loose, forcing you to start over. So keep it tight and braid close to the base of the bun.

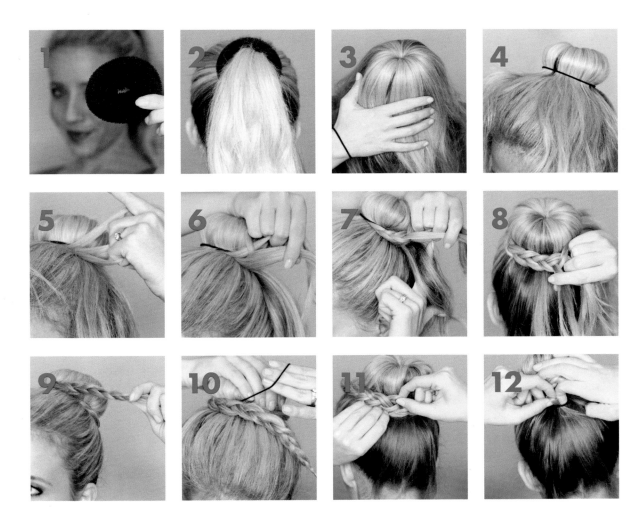

~Rope Bun~

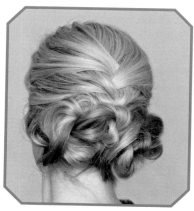

1. French Braid the hair along the center, going halfway down your head, and secure with a clear elastic band.

2. Split the remaining hair into two sections. Clip one section (you can see my purple clip holding the farther section). Split the remaining hair into two equal parts and twist each section in the same direction. It doesn't matter which direction, but they need to be twisting the same way.

3. Create a rope braid by twisting the two sections together in the opposite direction they were twisted in step 2 and secure with a clear elastic band.

4. Randomly pin the rope braid above to the nape of your neck. This is where you decide what shape you want and how you want the bun to look.

5. Repeat steps 2–4 on the other side making sure to mesh the buns together when you put up that second bun.

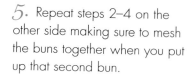

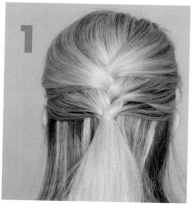

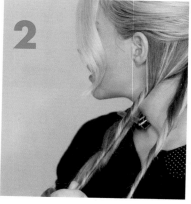

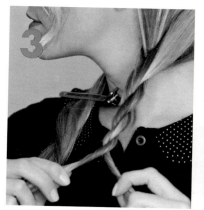

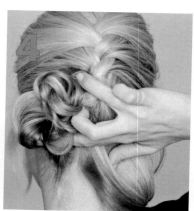

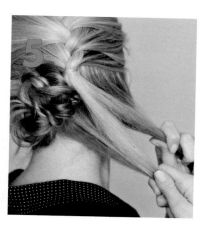

Knots

Knots are such a fun and flirty way to add texture and detail to a hairstyle. Everyone who sees your hair will be super impressed by these intricate creations. It'll be our little secret that they're much easier to do than they look! Just make sure when you're starting a knotted style that you either dampen your hair with water or have a tiny bit of a pomade or gel on your fingers to keep the frizz and flyaways at bay.

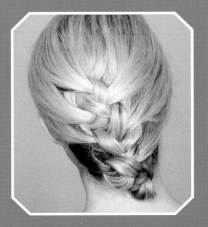
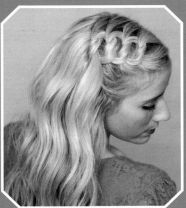
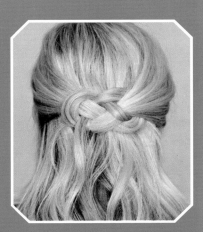

Knotted Bangs

Start this style with leftover 1-inch wand curls.

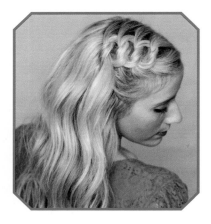

1. Take a 2-inch section of hair from the front and divide it in two sections.

2. Knot the two sections of hair by crossing the sections and bringing the bottom over and down through the hole.

3. Add a new section of hair to each side of the knot.

4. Knot the two sections. Cross the sections and bring the bottom over and down through the hole.

5. Repeat steps 3–4 until you have about four knots.

6. Take a bobby pin and insert it horizontally into the last knot. Use one bobby pin on each side of the knot, and the hair should easily cover up the pins.

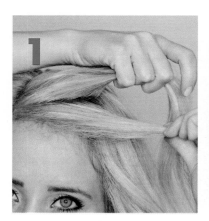
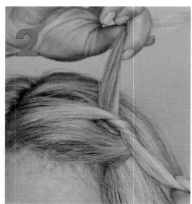
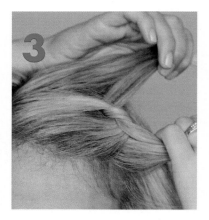
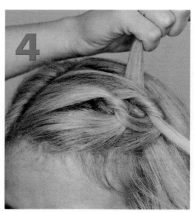
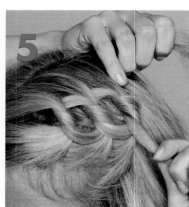
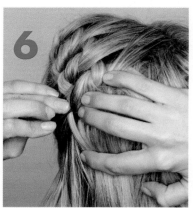

Hair Bow

What girl doesn't love bows? Seriously this hairstyle just makes me happy!

1-2. Brush your hair up into a nice high bun. Make sure to leave out about 3 to 4 inches of the ends on the last pass.

3. Split the bun in half.

4. Clip one side of the bun to your head with a duckbill clip.

5. Get your large bobby pins ready.

6. Attach the bun to your head by sliding the bobby pins in vertically. Repeat on other the side.

7. Bring the tail up and forward.

8. Bobby pin the tail near the base of the bun. Spray any flyaways down and pull out some fringe in the front to complete the look!

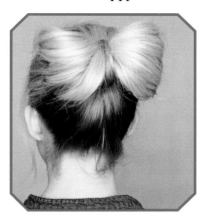

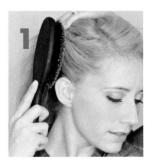
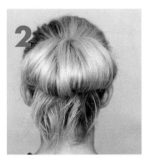
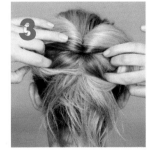
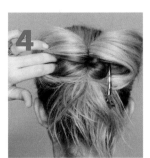

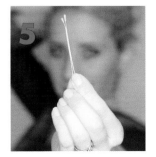
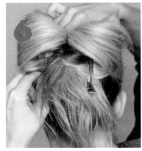
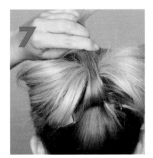
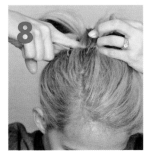

Knotty or Nice

1. Take two small sections of hair a few inches from the front.

2. Tie them in a knot below the crown of your head. It's important how you knot your hair in this style. You're going to cross the two sections and then bring the top section under and up.

3. Combine the tails and hold them with one hand. These tails will become half of the next knot.

4. With the other hand bring a section of hair back.

5. Tie a knot with the two sections, the one you just brought back and the one you made earlier. Remember to bring that top section under and up.

6. Add a small section of hair to each of the tails.

7. Combine the tails and gather a section of hair from the opposite side. Bring it back and tie it into another knot. Repeat these steps until you get to the nape of your neck.

8. Continue knotting the two sections of hair without adding new hair and tie off with a clear elastic band.

9. Roll the tail up and place it inside the small gap between the nape of your neck and the knotted style. If it doesn't feel secure, use a bobby pin to hold it in place.

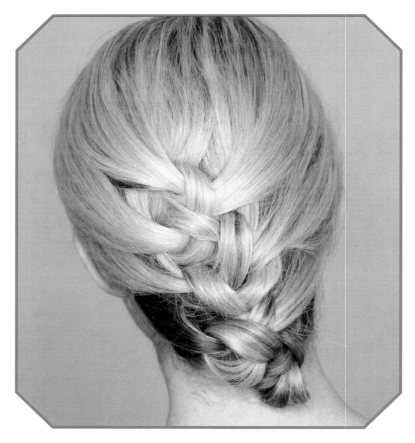

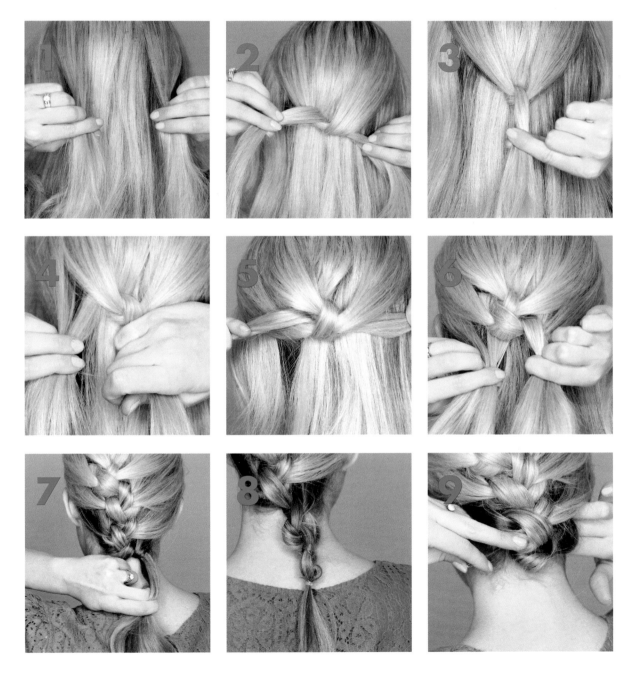

Celtic Knot

This is definitely the most difficult style in the book, but don't let that scare you away! Once you get it, the steps will be ingrained in your brain and it'll quickly become one of your *favorite* hairstyles. The compliments you'll get on this baby will have you crawling back for more!

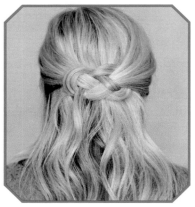

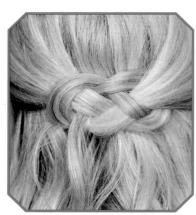

1. Take a section of hair from the left side and pull it back.

2. Wrap that section around two fingers on your left hand.

3. Continue wrapping until you form a loop. Slide your fingers out and hold that loop in your left hand. Pay attention to how I'm holding the loop. It's important that your fingers look exactly like mine.

4. While holding that loop you're going to grab another section of hair from the front on the right side.

5. Pull that section of hair back and place it between your pinky and ring finger on your left hand. We're going to call this Section A. You'll want to pull it very tightly as this next step can loosen it.

6. With your right hand, reach behind the front section of hair and pull up Section A.

7. Once you've pulled that section of hair up and over, take a duckbill clip and secure the loop. From here on out we're going to be working with Section A. If you've made it this far, the hardest steps are behind you.

8. Take Section A and thread it over and through the loop.

9. Now thread it underneath that front section of hair.

10. And back up through the bottom of the loop. Make sure to thread it from the back of the loop to the front.

11. Remove the duckbill clip, and pull the ends tight.

12. Finally, you're going to rearrange the knot and perfect it by sliding the knot around, pancaking some parts and tightening others. If you need to, pin behind the knot to secure it in place.

Before you begin, familiarize yourself with what the Celtic Knot looks like and make sure you have a second mirror handy. It really helps if you can see the back of your hair in a mirror without having to drop your hands to pick one up. We have a closet door in our bathroom that I've hung a mirror over, and when I open the door I can see the back of my hair through our vanity mirror. Being able to see the steps in the mirror and where the sections are will be extremely helpful.

I started this hairstyle with 1-inch wand curls (see pages 22–23).

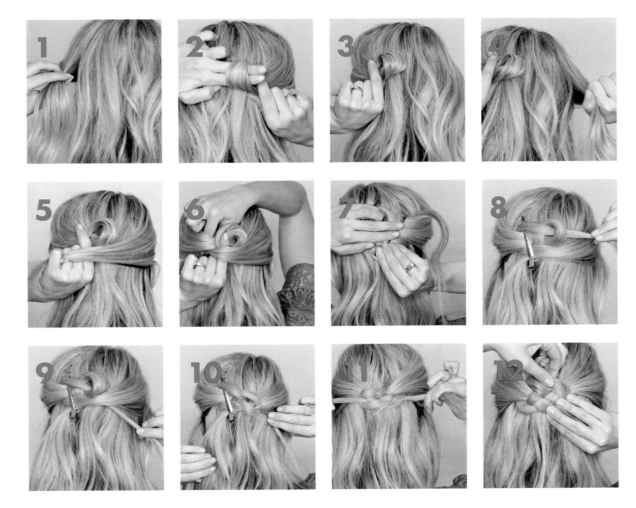

Half-Up Hair Bow

I started this hairstyle with 1-inch wand curls (see pages 22–23). This is a great style if you need to get that hair out of your face but want something that's still flirty and fun!

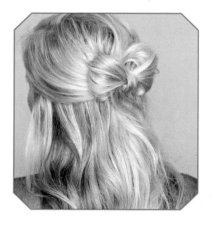

1. Gather the hair from above your ears up into a simple half bun. Make sure to leave out a few inches of the ends as we need them to finish the style.

2. Split the bun into two sections.

3. Use a duckbill clip to secure one of the sections.

4. Insert a bobby pin in vertically to hold the bow in place. Remove the clip and repeat on the other side.

5. Take half of the ends you left out and bring them up.

6. Pull them through the bow with the other hand.

7. Secure them with bobby pins and repeat with the other half on the other side of the bow.

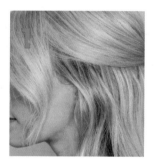
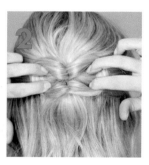
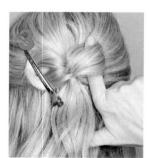
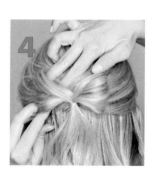

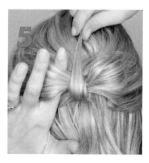
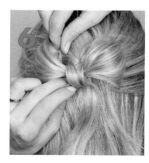
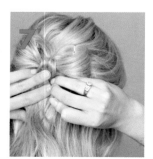

Twists

Twists are gorgeous. They have such pretty and elegant shapes, and they can easily be pancaked to add great texture to any style. I love experimenting with all the different types of twists, and honestly the possibilities are endless! If you know your basic braids and twists, you can do anything you want with your hair. Use one braid as a base and add a twist . . . and another! By layering styles you'll create gorgeous 'dos that are uniquely you. If you come up with a new twist hairstyle all your own, I'd love to see it! Tag photos of your braids to @twistmepretty on Instagram.

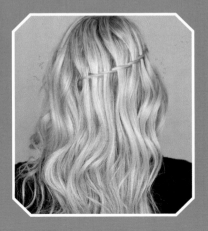
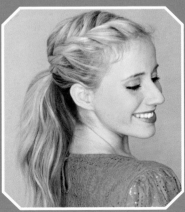
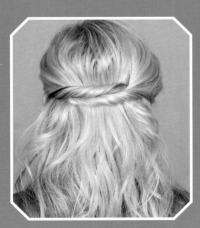

ᏊTwisted HaloᏊ

This hairstyle looks very similar to a regular Bohemian Twist, however it's a little bit different. Basically you'll be twisting the sections on the heavy side toward the face instead of away and adding in new hair only to the back sections of the twist.

1. Give yourself a deep side part. I like to use the outside corners of my eyebrows as a guide. Take a 1-inch section of hair and divide it into two equal sections.

2. Twist the back section forward and over the front section.

3. Combine both sections into your back hand. The front section will be held by your index finger and thumb and the back section by your pinky and ring fingers. Take your free hand and add a new section of hair to that back section, the one held by your pinky and ring fingers.

4. Twist the sections forward.

5. Continue twisting and adding in hair until the twist reaches a few inches behind your temples. Continue twisting until you run out of hair.

6. Gently drape the twist around the back of your head and secure with a duckbill clip.

7. Take a large section of hair from the front on the other side and split into two sections. Twist the bottom section over the top section. Add hair to the top section and the bottom section and twist up. Continue with just a regular two-strand twist (without adding any hair) through the length of the hair.

8. Angle the twist around your head. Tie it off with a clear elastic band.

9. Wrap that twist as far as it will go around along your first twist and secure it with a bobby pin behind the first twist.

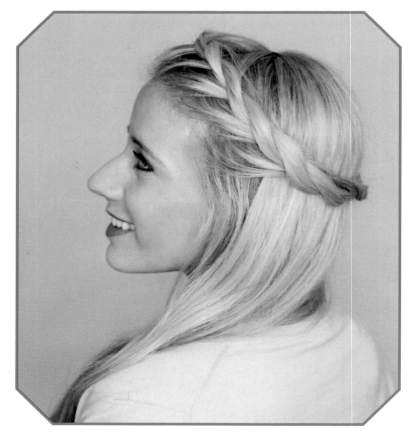

10. Remove the duckbill clip and secure the hair behind the second twist with a bobby pin. If needed, pancake the twist to make it look fuller and more voluminous.

Tip

I added a few curls into my hair with a 1.25-inch wand, compressed the curls in my hand until they were cool, then released them and fingered through. Finish this style off with a firm-hold hair spray!

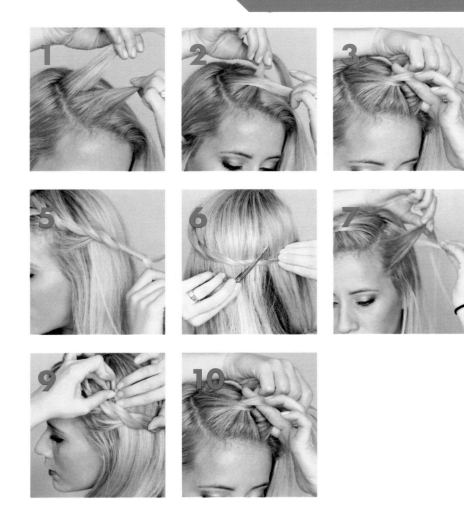

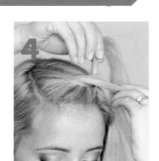

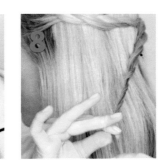

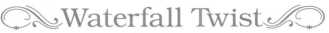

Waterfall Twist

Start by curling the hair with a 1-inch wand (see pages 22–23).

1. Take a triangular section of hair from the front and divide it into two sections. Combine the sections into the front hand.

2. With your back hand, gather a new section of hair from near your part and behind the front section. You want this new section to be equal in size to the other two.

3. Drop the new section in between the two original sections.

4. Take the two original sections and twist them up, the bottom section going over the top section. To tighten the waterfall'ing sections, pull them taut.

5. Gather a new section of hair from near your part and drop it through the center of the two original sections. Twist them up.

6. Repeat steps 2–5, wrapping the twist as far as it will go around the crown of your head. Secure it by sliding a bobby pin in through the twists.

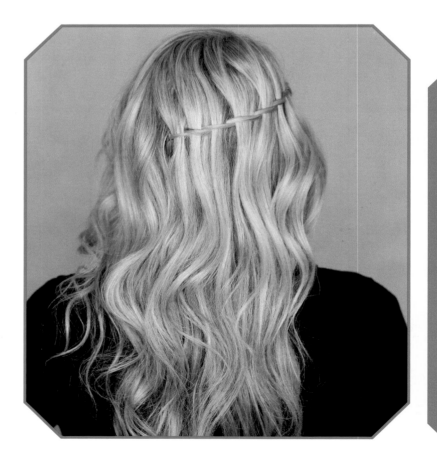

My front sections of hair are not as long as the back, and because I'm twisting those original two sections all the way back, I've gone as far as the length would reach. If you have hair to keep twisting, keep going! It'd be super cute to twist all the way to the front and down like in the Waterfall Braid on pages 42–43.

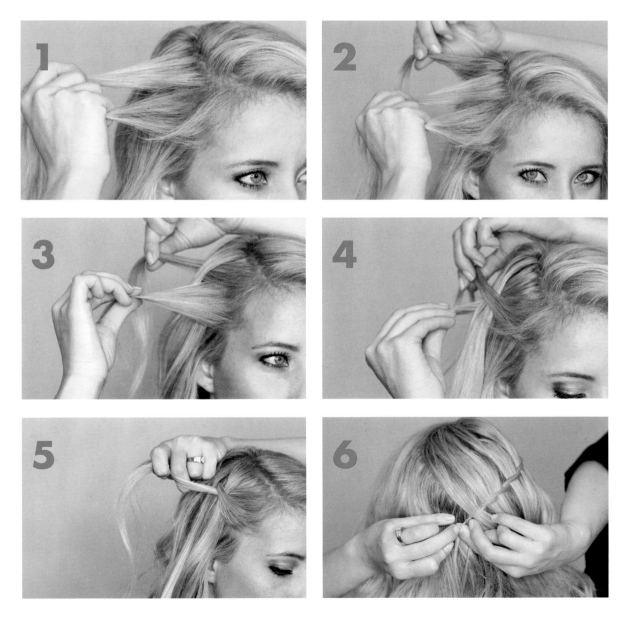

Waterfall Flower

I added this hairstyle to the book because 1, it's really cute, but 2, I feel like it's a perfect example of how easy it is to build braids and twists onto each other. I started by curling my hair with a 1-inch wand. You'll be braiding a Waterfall Twist so if you need in-depth instructions visit pages 112–113.

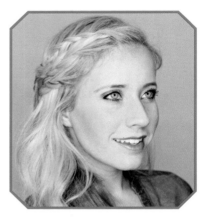

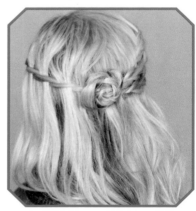

1. Split a triangular section near your part into two sections.

2. Move the sections into the front hand, and with your back hand grab another equal section of hair.

3. Drop that section in between the two original sections and twist up the two original sections.

4. Continue twisting until you've reached three or four inches behind your temples. Secure the hair by sliding a bobby pin into the twists.

5. Repeat steps 1–4 on the other side until you reach the first twist.

6. Take a small chunk of hair from the front and do a regular three-strand braid all the way back.

7. Secure the braid where it meets the twists with a clear elastic band.

8. Now take a chunk of hair from where all the twists and braids meet and braid a regular three-strand braid all the way down the length of the hair.

9. Begin rolling the braid.

10. Discretely pin the braid in place and you've created a nice little flower!

This style started with a Waterfall Twist, and then I wasn't getting the exact shape I wanted, so I added a regular three-strand braid and arranged the ends into a little flower. Play around with your hair, and feel free to create new styles! If you've spent time braiding your hair and you're just not loving it, don't just undo it. Add to it, fix the shape, and get creative!

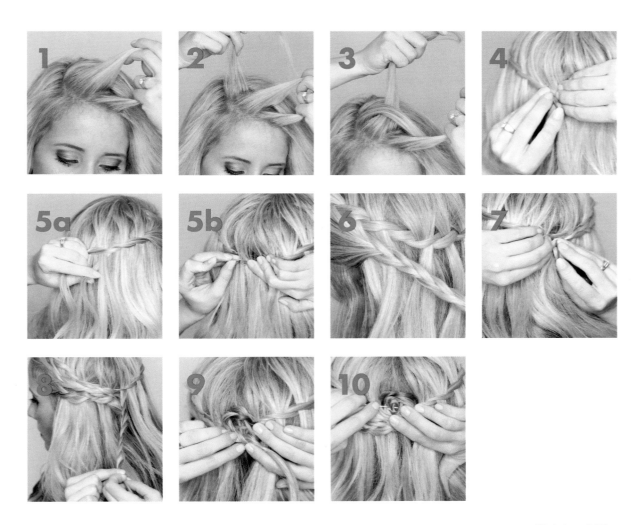

Bohemian Twist Ponytail

This style uses the Falling Bohemian Twist technique. If you need to familiarize yourself with that hairstyle you can find it on pages 32–33.

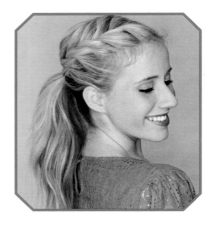

1. Divide a small section of hair near your part into two separate sections.

2. Twist the bottom over the top section.

3. Add in hair to the top section, just like you would with a French Braid, and add hair to the bottom section. Twist the sections up.

4. Continue to wrap the twist around to the back of your head, and secure it with a duckbill clip.

5. Repeat steps 1–5 on the other side by dividing hair into two equal sections.

6. Twist them up.

7. Add hair to the top section and to the bottom section.

8. Twist up.

9. Continue twisting the hair around your head.

10. Once the twists meet, release the duckbill clip of the first twist and secure the hairstyle into a ponytail with a clear elastic band.

Tip

I find it helpful to take the end of a rattail comb and push it through the hair a few inches from the roots. Gently lift up on the comb to add more volume to the hairstyle and really polish off the look.

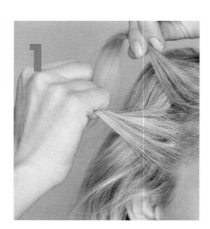

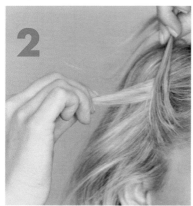

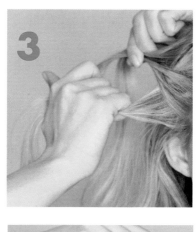

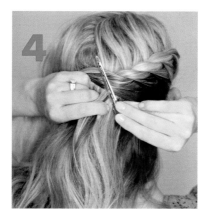

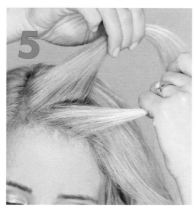

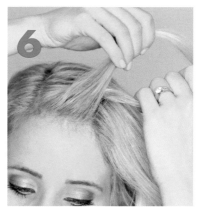

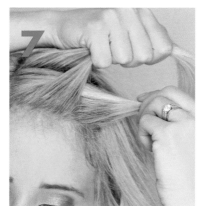

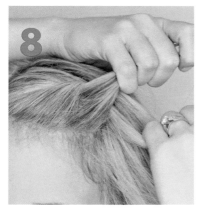

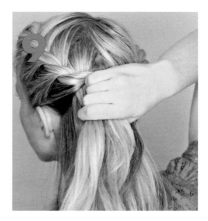

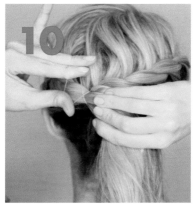

~Twisted Together~

Start this style by teasing the roots and curling with a 1-inch wand (see pages 22–23).

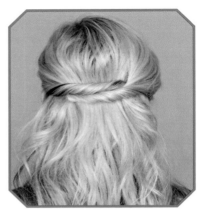

1. Gather the front section of hair and loosely twist it back. I am twisting the hair away from my face, but you can go in either direction.

2. To pancake the twist, hold the end of the twist tight with one hand and with the other hand loosen the areas of the twist that you'd like to be fuller.

3. Slide a bobby pin in horizontally.

4. Repeat steps 1–2 on the opposite side. Drape the new twist directly above the first twist.

5. Slide the top twist behind the first twist and pin with a bobby pin or two.

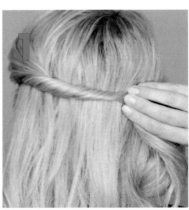

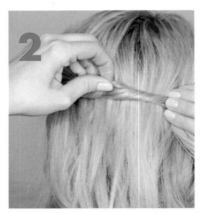

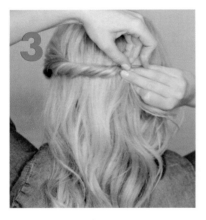

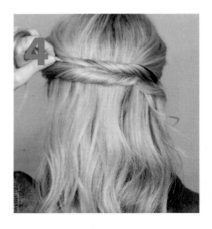

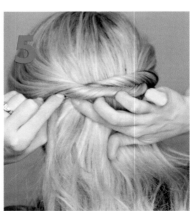

Topsy Tails

Well, well, well, what do we have here?! Do you remember the Topsy Tail from when you were a little girl? The style is back, and I'm here to throw a modern twist on it. There are so many amazing things you can do with a Topsy Tail, so make sure you know what it is and how to make it!

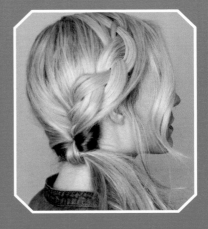

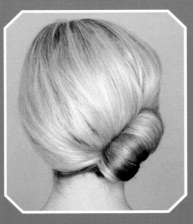

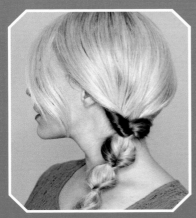

Simple Topsy Tail

Here's how to make a Topsy Tail without using the styling tool. You can use this for any of the Topsy Tail styles in this book.

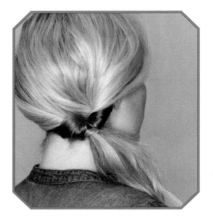

1. Gather your hair into a low side ponytail.

2. Gently slide the elastic down a couple of inches. Divide the hair with your fingers and make a hole directly above the elastic.

3. Now flip the tail up and through the hole. To get that pretty shape, you'll need to split the ponytail into two sections and pull, cinching up the elastic and tightening the Topsy Tail.

Tip

Instead of making a Topsy Tail manually you can purchase a Topsy Tail styling tool. They are very easy to use and are super cheap. I would definitely get one!

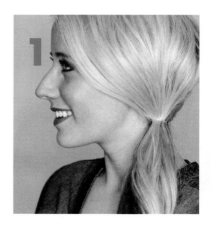

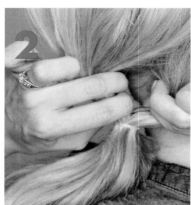

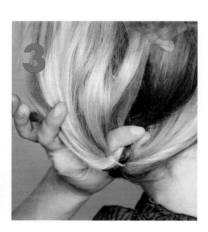

Topsy Tail Faux Fishtail

You're going to start by putting your hair into a side Topsy Tail. This style is basically a succession of Topsy Tails and so simple it's even dad-friendly!

1. Tie a clear elastic band a few inches down from the first Topsy Tail.

2. Slide your Topsy Tail styling tool into the hair right above the elastic. Pull your ponytail through the opening at the top of the Topsy Tail tool and then pull down on the Topsy Tail tool. This is going to flip your ponytail inside the hole and create that really pretty style.

3. You may need to cinch up on the elastic band to get that perfect shape. You can do that by dividing the tail into two sections and pulling.

4. Continue adding as many Topsy Tails as the hair length allows. To make the Fishtail fuller, pull out and tug on the pieces. Even a Topsy Tail can be pancaked!

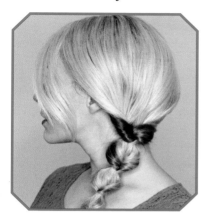

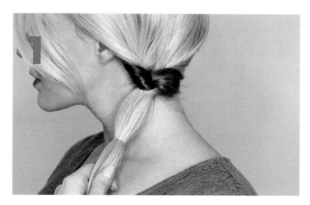

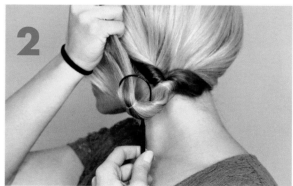

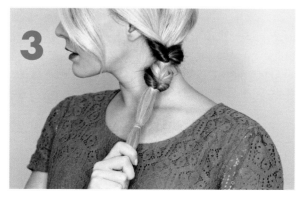

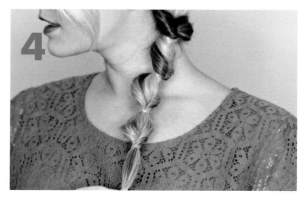

Dutch Braided Topsy Tail

This is a great third- or fourth-day hairstyle, especially when you have really loose waves from leftover curls.

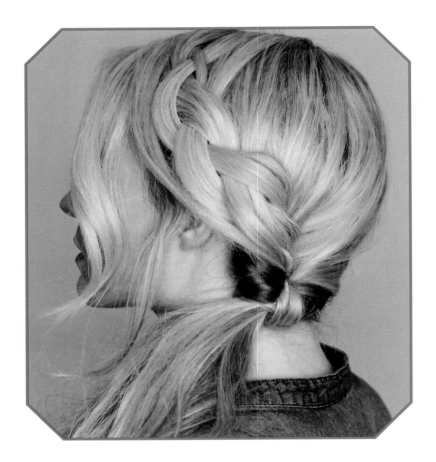

1-2. Section off some hair in the front, and pull the rest of your hair into a low side ponytail. Then simply put it into a Topsy Tail. If you don't have a Topsy Tail tool, make a hole above the elastic with your fingers and pull the ponytail up and through it.

3. Take the section of hair you left out and throw it back in a Dutch French Braid. Feel free to leave out your bangs or pull them all back.

4. Braid all the way down and secure with a clear elastic band.

5. Pancake the braid by spreading apart the layers.

6. Reach your finger up through the hole you made when you created the Topsy Tail and pull the braid through. Tease the ponytail and finish off with hair spray.

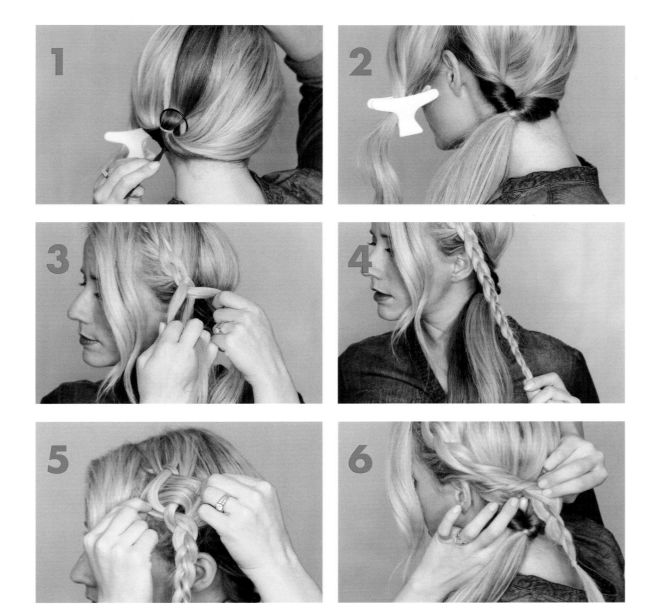

Topsy Tail Chignon

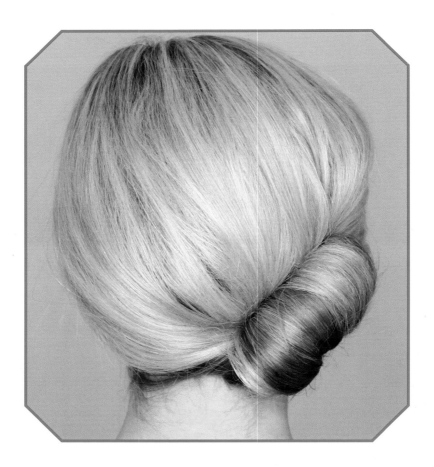

1–2. Put your hair into a side Topsy Tail.

3. Reach up through the hole of your Topsy Tail and pull the ponytail ends through the hole.

4. If you still have length left, repeat step 3 by pushing the hair through the hole of the Topsy Tail and grabbing underneath it with your index finger to hide the ends. Spray with a firm-hold hair spray in the direction your hair is moving.

5. Now take a large bobby pin and thread it through the chignon. This is going to ensure the style holds, and it will also give lift to the bun.

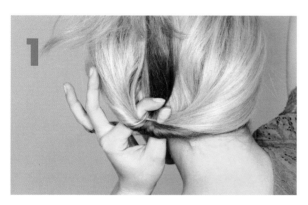

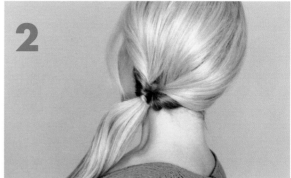

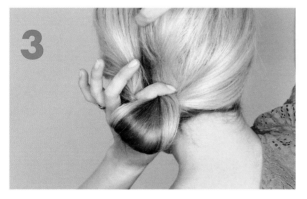

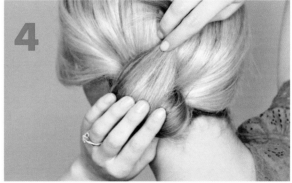

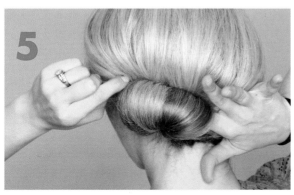

Layered Topsy Tails

This is such a fun ponytail, and it only requires a few extra steps! Start by curling the hair with a 1-inch wand (see pages 22–23). and teasing the roots.

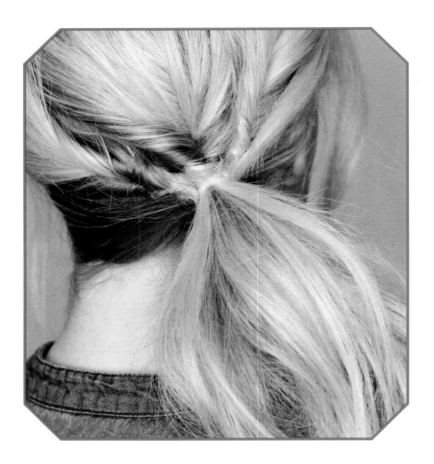

1. Gather a small section of hair near the front and tie it off with a clear elastic band.

2. Create a Topsy Tail out of that section either by using a Topsy Tail styling tool or by making a hole right above the elastic . . .

3. . . . and flipping the tail through it. Make sure you're angling all the Topsy Tails toward where you want your final ponytail to sit.

4. Take another section from the back and make a Topsy Tail.

5. Gather a third and final section from the other side of your head and make another Topsy Tail. Pull all the ends into a low side ponytail and secure it with a clear elastic band.

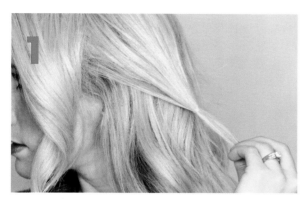

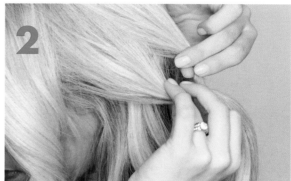

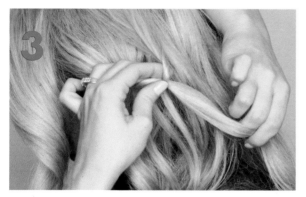

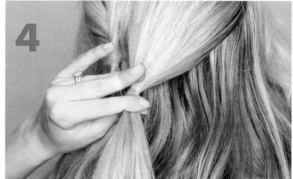

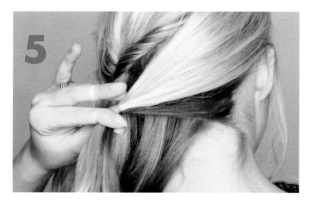

Tip

These Topsy Tails don't need to be super tight; in fact they'll look prettier if they have more volume and are a little bit loose.

Wrapped Ponytail

I'm sure you've wrapped a small section of hair around your ponytail before. You probably pinned it with a bobby pin, and hours later you've found that the wrap is randomly sticking out and the bobby pin is nowhere to be found. Well don't worry; I've got your back!

1. Pull your hair up into a ponytail, then wrap the entire tail around a hot 1.25-inch curling wand.

2. Gently slide the wand out and quickly wrap the hair around your fingers in the same direction you had it wrapped around the wand.

3. Compress the hair by flattening the curl in between your hands. This is going to set the curl and give you a gorgeous shape in the ponytail. Once the curl is cool, release it. Tease the ponytail and scrunch up the curls with your hand while spraying with a firm-hold hair spray.

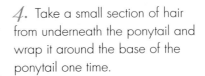

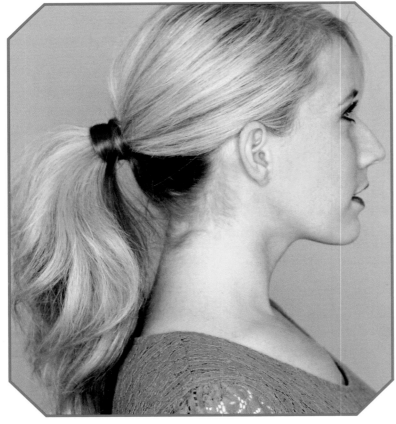

4. Take a small section of hair from underneath the ponytail and wrap it around the base of the ponytail one time.

5. Take a Topsy Tail styling tool and insert it right above the elastic band. Put the section of hair you're wrapping through the tool's opening.

6. Pull on the Topsy Tail tool and your small section of hair will come out at the bottom of your ponytail. Continue wrapping that section around the hair and threading it through the Topsy Tail tool until you've run out of hair to thread. This is going to secure that section of hair without the use of any bobby pins and it's going to look very effortless and natural.

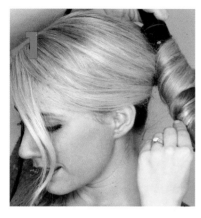
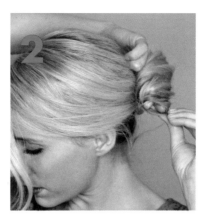
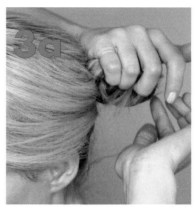
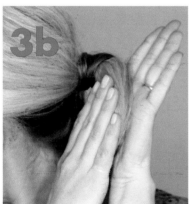
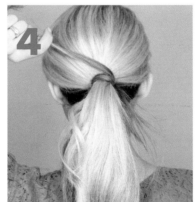
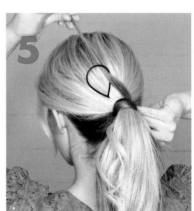
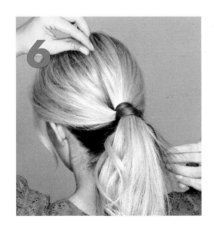

Topsy Tail Messy Bun

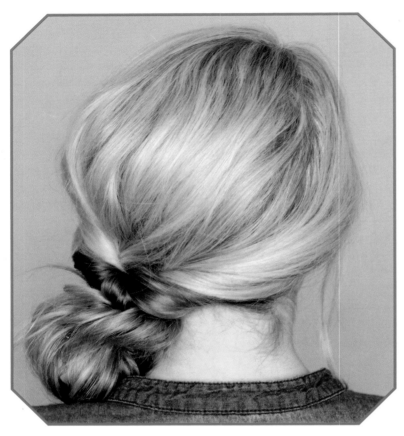

1. Put the hair into a side Topsy Tail. Refer to tutorial on page 120.

2. Create a Fast Messy Bun directly below the Topsy Tail by pulling your ponytail into a new elastic right underneath the Topsy Tail and following the steps on pages 92–93.

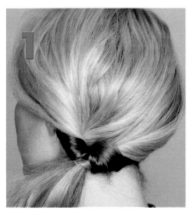

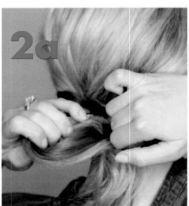

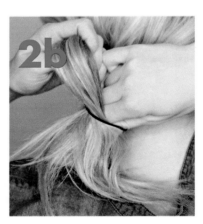

Topsy Tail High Bun

1. Start by pulling your hair into a high ponytail. Then create a Topsy Tail by reaching through the front of the elastic.

2. Grabbing the ponytail.

3. And pulling it up.

4. Holding the ponytail up, tease the ponytail with a rattail comb and finger through any snarls.

5. Take the ends of your ponytail and push them up through the Topsy Tail hole. If you need to secure the bun even further, take a couple of large bobby pins and insert one onto each side of the bun. Finish by pulling out bangs and fringe and spraying with hair spray.

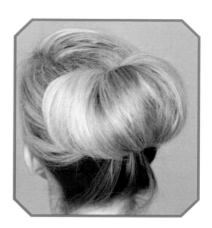

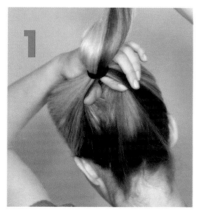

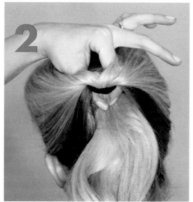

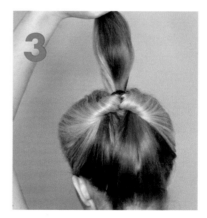

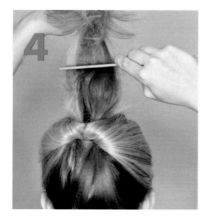

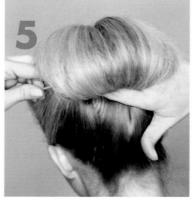

Index

About the Author

Abby Smith is a happily married mother of two. She and her family live in Orem, Utah, where her husband is finishing his education at Brigham Young University. Her desire to be a stay-at-home mother and her passion for beauty and blogging compelled her to create the popular website *Twist Me Pretty*.

Abby is the author of *The Ultimate Hairstyle Handbook*, is a beauty expert for Disney's own Babble.com, and loves to create and inspire women of all ages to feel beautiful and confident in their own skin. For video tutorials on even more styles than the ones you find in this book, check out her You-Tube channel: http://www.youtube.com/user/twistmepretty.

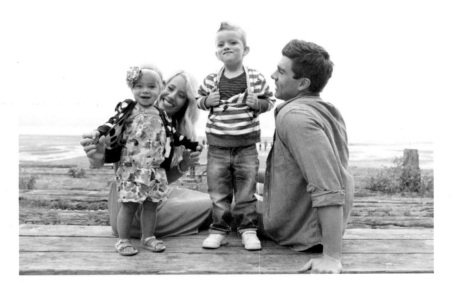